The Science of Muscular Strength

The Science of Muscular Strength

Rafeal Mechlore

UNIEK ENTERPRISES

CONTENTS

INDEX

INTRODUCTION

Solid strength is a major part of human physiology that has enraptured the interest of researchers, competitors, and wellbeing devotees for quite a long time. It addresses the limit of our muscles to produce power and assumes a significant part in our regular routines, from the least complex errands like lifting a staple pack to the most requesting athletic accomplishments, like Olympic weightlifting. The quest for more prominent strong strength has been a main impetus behind innumerable preparation regimens, dietary plans, and, surprisingly, the improvement of state of the art innovations. A point incorporates the physical as well as the mental and physiological elements of human life.

In this thorough investigation of "The Study of Solid Strength," we set out on an excursion through the perplexing trap of elements that impact our capacity to produce force, from the sub-atomic systems inside our muscle filaments to the unpredictable brain processes interfacing cerebrum and sturdiness. Throughout this 2000-word venture, we will dive into the logical underpinnings of strong strength, addressing points like muscle physiology, brain transformations, preparing techniques, dietary contemplations, and the more extensive ramifications for wellbeing and execution.

The Authentic Mission for Strength

The human interest with strong strength can be followed back to old times, where legends of godlike strength and legends have large amounts of folklores from around the world. Whether it was Hercules in Greek folklore, Samson in the Jewish Book of scriptures, or endless other social symbols, these accounts frequently celebrated and mythologized the exceptional capacities of solidarity.

In the later past, the mission for strength developed from fanciful stories to logical requests. The nineteenth and twentieth hundreds of years saw spearheading work by physiologists and researchers like August Krogh, Archibald V. Slope, and H.G. Wells, who established the groundworks for our advanced comprehension of strong strength. Their exploration investigated the components behind muscle constriction, energy creation, and the job of nerves in organizing muscle movement.

Muscle Physiology: The Driving force of Solidarity

At the core of the study of solid strength lies muscle physiology. Muscles, the workhorses of the body, are perplexing designs made out of muscle strands that agreement because of brain signals. To comprehend strong strength, we should analyze the infinitesimal world inside our muscles.

Muscle constriction is essentially fueled by the sliding fiber hypothesis. It includes the communication between two proteins, actin and myosin, which slide past one another to abbreviate the muscle fiber. This interaction consumes adenosine tri-phosphate (ATP),

the energy money of cells. The more noteworthy the power required, the more muscle strands are enrolled, bringing about more grounded constrictions.

Muscle filaments are not no different either way; they can be sorted into slow-jerk (Type I) and quick jerk (Type II) strands. Type I strands are adjusted for perseverance and produce less power yet can contract for broadened periods. Then again, Type II strands are specific for fast, strong constrictions however weakness all the more rapidly. The creation of these fiber types inside a singular's muscles assumes a basic part in deciding their innate strength potential.

Brain Variations: The Psyche Muscle Association

Strong strength isn't exclusively about the muscle filaments themselves; it's simi-larly reliant upon the sensory system's capacity to actually enlist and direction these strands. This is where the idea of neuromuscular transformation becomes urgent.

The focal sensory system, especially the cerebrum and spinal string, assumes a sig-nificant part in controlling muscle withdrawals. At the point when you choose to lift a weighty item, your cerebrum conveys messages through engine neurons to initiate the pertinent muscle strands. With preparing and practice, these brain connections become more productive, taking into consideration more noteworthy synchroniza-tion and enrollment of muscle filaments - a peculiarity known as brain variation.

Moreover, engine units, which comprise of an engine neuron and the muscle filaments it innervates, can be specifically selected relying upon the power required. At first, the more modest, slow-jerk engine units are locked in for lighter errands, however as the interest for strength increments, bigger, quick jerk engine units are enrolled. This enlistment design is finely tuned through training and preparing, eventually adding to a singular's solidarity potential.

Preparing Systems: Fashioning Solid Strength

The mission for more prominent solid strength is a main thrust behind different preparation strategies and ways of thinking. From powerlifting to working out, from exercises to Olympic weightlifting, there are innumerable ways of developing forti-tude, each with its extraordinary standards and preparing methods.

Obstruction preparing, which includes lifting loads or utilizing opposition groups, is a typical way to deal with developing strong fortitude. Moderate over-burden, a cen-tral rule, involves continuously expanding the protection from persistently challenge the muscles. Compound developments like squats, deadlifts, and seat presses draw in different muscle gatherings and are frequently at the center of solidarity building programs.

The recurrence, power, and volume of instructional courses all assume a basic part in deciding the results of a strength-preparing program. In addition, periodization, the deliberate variety of preparing factors after some time, forestalls levels and improve strength gains.

Healthful Contemplations: Energizing the Fire

Muscles, similar to some other hardware, require appropriate fuel to ideally work. Nourishment is a key part of the study of solid strength. The macronutrients - carbs, proteins, and fats - give the energy and building blocks fundamental for muscle development and fix.

Starches are the body's essential energy source, providing the ATP required for muscle constrictions. Protein, made out of amino acids, is fundamental for muscle fix and development. Dietary fat, while frequently neglected, assumes a urgent part in chemical creation and generally wellbeing, by implication influencing strength improvement.

Besides, micronutrients like nutrients and minerals add to different physiological cycles that influence strong strength. For example, calcium is fundamental for muscle compression, while vitamin D assumes a part in muscle capability and bone wellbeing. An even eating routine that meets the particular necessities of solidarity competitors is fundamental for streamlining execution and recuperation.

Past Games: Solid Strength and Wellbeing

While solid strength is frequently connected with athletic execution and weight training, its significance stretches out a long ways past these pursuits. It is a vital part of generally speaking wellbeing and prosperity, with suggestions for everyday exercises and long haul personal satisfaction.

Keeping up with strong strength is especially significant as we age. Sarcopenia, the age-related loss of bulk and strength, can prompt decreased versatility, expanded chance of falls, and a lower personal satisfaction. Strength preparing, even in later years, has been displayed to balance these impacts, protecting utilitarian autonomy and advancing life span.

Furthermore, solid strength straightforwardly affects metabolic wellbeing. Muscle tissue is metabolically dynamic, meaning it consumes calories even very still. Expanded bulk can assist with managing blood glucose levels, further develop insulin awareness, and diminish the gamble of metabolic problems like sort 2 diabetes.

Chapter 1

Defining Muscular Strength

Solid strength is a basic part of actual wellness and assumes a critical part in our regular routines. It's the capacity of your muscles to create force against opposition, and it includes different parts of actual execution. This paper digs profound into the idea of solid strength, investigating its definition, significance, estimation, factors influencing it, and procedures for its turn of events.

Characterizing Solid Strength

Solid strength can be characterized as the greatest measure of power a muscle or a gathering of muscles can produce in a solitary, full scale exertion. It is many times estimated in units of power, like pounds or kilograms. This definition recognizes strong strength from different parts of wellness, for example, solid perseverance, which alludes to the capacity to support submaximal compressions over a drawn out period.

Solid strength isn't uniform all through the body; different muscle bunches display fluctuating degrees of solidarity. For instance, the muscles of the legs, like the quadriceps and hamstrings, will generally be more grounded than those in the chest area, like the biceps and rear arm muscles. Also, individual contrasts in strength can exist because of hereditary qualities, preparing history, and different elements.

Significance of Solid Strength

Practical Capacities: Solid strength is fundamental for performing regular exercises, for example, lifting food, climbing steps, or pushing a weighty item. Without adequate strength, these assignments become seriously testing and can prompt actual constraints.

Injury Anticipation: Solid muscles give dependability and backing to joints, diminishing the gamble of injury. A solid center, for example, can assist with keeping up with legitimate stance and safeguard the spine during lifting and different developments.

Improved Athletic Execution: In sports and athletic undertakings, solid strength is in many cases a deciding variable. Competitors expect solidarity to run quicker, hop higher, toss farther, and contend at their most elevated level.

Metabolic Advantages: Building and keeping up with bulk can increment digestion, prompting more proficient calorie consuming and possibly supporting weight the board and fat misfortune.

Improving with age: As we age, bulk normally declines, bringing about diminished strength and portability. Ordinary strength preparing can relieve these impacts, permitting people to keep up with autonomy and personal satisfaction as they progress in years.

Estimating Strong Strength

One-Reiteration Greatest (1RM): This is the most broadly involved strategy for evaluating strong strength. It includes deciding the most extreme weight an individual can lift for a solitary redundancy of a given activity, for example, seat press, squat, or deadlift.

Isometric Testing: In isometric strength testing, the muscle contracts against a decent opposition, yet there is no apparent development. Gadgets like dynamometers and handgrip strength analyzers are usually utilized for isometric strength appraisals.

Isokinetic Testing: Isokinetic testing estimates strength through a scope of movement at a consistent speed. Particular hardware is expected for this kind of testing, which is in many cases utilized in recovery settings.

Practical Testing: Useful tests survey strong strength by assessing a singular's capacity to perform explicit errands, for example, push-ups, pull-ups, or sit-ups. These tests give a reasonable proportion of solidarity in exercises pertinent to day to day existence.

Electromyography (EMG): EMG estimates the electrical action of muscles during withdrawal. While not an immediate proportion of solidarity, it gives important bits of knowledge into muscle enlistment designs and can be utilized to survey muscle weakness.

Biodex Testing: Biodex machines are utilized to assess strength, perseverance, and power through isokinetic testing. They are much of the time utilized in research and clinical settings.

Factors Influencing Solid Strength

Hereditary qualities: Hereditary inclination assumes a critical part in a singular's true capacity for strong strength. Certain individuals may normally have a more prominent ability to fabricate and keep up with bulk.

Preparing: Moderate obstruction preparing is the best method for expanding strong strength. Ordinary exercises that challenge muscles to adjust and become stronger turn of events.

Nourishment: Sufficient protein admission is pivotal for muscle development and fix. Appropriate nourishment gives the structure blocks important to muscle improvement.

Chemicals: Chemicals, for example, testosterone and development chemical assume fundamental parts in muscle development and strength improvement. Hormonal lopsided characteristics can influence strength gains.

Age: Muscle strength will in general top in youthful adulthood and bit by bit decline with age. Nonetheless, opposition preparing can assist with moderating age-related strength misfortune.

Sex: by and large, men will generally have more prominent bulk and strength contrasted with ladies, essentially because of hormonal contrasts. Nonetheless, ladies can in any case accomplish critical strength acquires through preparing.

Recuperation: Muscles need satisfactory rest and recuperation time to fix and develop further. Overtraining can prompt muscle exhaustion and obstruct strength gains.

Neuromuscular Transformations: Upgrades in strong strength are not exclusively because of muscle size yet additionally include brain variations. Better coordination and muscle enrollment examples can upgrade strength.

Procedures for Creating Solid Strength

Obstruction Preparing: Participate in an organized opposition preparing program that objectives significant muscle gatherings. Utilize free loads, machines, obstruction groups, or bodyweight activities to give moderate opposition.

Moderate Over-burden: Constantly increment the obstruction or power of your exercises to challenge your muscles and animate development. Slow movement is critical to progressing strength gains.

Appropriate Structure: Keep up with legitimate method during activities to decrease the gamble of injury and guarantee that you're focusing on the planned muscle bunches really.

Variety: Incorporate different activities to work all significant muscle gatherings and forestall levels. This can likewise assist with forestalling abuse wounds.

Rest and Recuperation: Permit muscles satisfactory chance to recuperate between exercises. This is when muscle fix and development happen.

Sustenance: Consume a reasonable eating routine wealthy in protein to help muscle fix and development. Appropriate hydration is likewise fundamental.

Consistency: Consistency is significant in strength preparing. Go for the gold, preferably 2-4 times each week, to see critical upgrades.

Periodization: Integrate periodization into your preparation plan, which includes modifying the power and volume of your exercises over the long run to keep away from stagnation.

Supplementation: Think about supplementation with protein, creatine, or different mixtures that might uphold muscle development and recuperation. Counsel a medical services proficient prior to beginning any enhancements.

Recuperation Methodologies: Use recuperation procedures, for example, extending, froth rolling, and back rub to decrease muscle irritation and further develop adaptability.

Counsel an Expert: In the event that you're new to strength preparing or have explicit objectives, consider working with an ensured fitness coach who can plan a tweaked program and give direction on legitimate procedure.

1.1 Importance in Everyday Life and Sports

Strong strength, the capacity of muscles to create force against opposition, holds colossal importance in both day to day existence and sports. A fundamental component of actual wellness impacts our capacity to perform different undertakings and succeed in athletic undertakings. In this thorough investigation, we will dive into the significance of strong strength in regular day to day existence and sports, featuring its effect on wellbeing, usefulness, and athletic execution.

Regular daily existence: The Groundwork of Usefulness

Utilitarian Undertakings: Solid strength is urgent for performing routine exercises, like lifting weighty articles, conveying food, and moving furnishings. Without sufficient strength, these errands can become testing and even lead to wounds.

Autonomy: As people age, keeping up with solid strength turns out to be significantly more basic. Solid muscles support versatility, balance, and the capacity to freely perform exercises of day to day living. Older people with great strong strength are more averse to encounter falls and cracks.

Stance and Spinal Wellbeing: Solid center muscles, including the abs and lower back muscles, assume a fundamental part in keeping up with legitimate stance and supporting the spine. A solid center forestalls conditions like lower back torment and works on in general spinal wellbeing.

Bone Wellbeing: Obstruction preparing, a critical part of solid strength improvement, can decidedly influence bone thickness. This is especially significant for people in danger of osteoporosis, as more grounded bones are stronger to cracks.

Metabolic Wellbeing: Building and keeping up with bulk through strength preparing can help digestion. Muscles consume a larger number of calories very still than fat, possibly helping with weight the executives and decreasing the gamble of heftiness related medical problems.

Joint: Serious areas of strength for soundness give steadiness to joints, diminishing the gamble of wounds and conditions like osteoarthritis. Appropriately molded muscles assist with conveying powers all the more uniformly, safeguarding the joints.

Torment Anticipation: Solid irregular characteristics and shortcomings can prompt different types of agony, for example, knee torment, hip agony, and shoulder torment. Fortifying the significant muscle gatherings can ease or forestall such distress.

Sports: An Upper hand

Athletic Execution: Strong strength is a crucial part of athletic execution in different games. It straightforwardly impacts a competitor's capacity to run quicker, hop higher, toss farther, and contend at their most elevated level.

Speed and Power: Dangerous developments, such as running, major areas of strength for require muscles to produce fast power against the ground. Competitors with more prominent strong strength can speed up more rapidly and accomplish higher velocities.

Hopping skill: Strong strength in the lower body, especially the quadriceps and lower leg muscles, is fundamental for bouncing games like b-ball and volleyball. A solid leg drive permits competitors to jump higher and with more control.

High-intensity games: Even in high-intensity games like cycling and significant distance running, strong strength assumes a basic part.

Solid leg muscles can keep a predictable speed and oppose weakness overstretched distances.

Injury Avoidance: Strength preparing can assist with forestalling sports-related wounds by improving joint solidness, muscle equilibrium, and generally speaking flexibility. Competitors with advanced muscles are less inclined to strains, injuries, and abuse wounds.

Sport-Explicit Developments: Many games require explicit muscle gatherings to succeed. For example, swimmers depend serious areas of strength for on body muscles, while gymnasts need outstanding center and chest area strength for soundness and control.

Recuperation and Restoration: Strong strength is important in the recovery cycle after sports wounds. Solid muscles support the mending system and assist competitors with getting back to their game all the more rapidly.

Strategic Benefit: In physical games like football and rugby, strong strength gives a strategic benefit. More grounded players can overwhelm truly, making it trying for rivals to guard or handle actually.

Estimation and Appraisal

To see the value in the significance of strong strength in both regular day to day existence and sports, it's fundamental to comprehend how it very well may be estimated and surveyed.

One-Reiteration Greatest (1RM): This generally utilized technique includes deciding the most extreme weight an individual can lift for a solitary redundancy of a particular activity, for example, the seat press or squat. 1RM testing is normal in sports preparing and can uncover a competitor's standard strength.

Utilitarian Testing: For regular day to day existence applications, useful tests survey strong strength by assessing one's capacity to perform down to earth undertakings. Models incorporate the capacity to convey a weighty burden up a stairwell or complete a set number of push-ups or squats.

Isokinetic Testing: Isokinetic testing estimates strength through a scope of movement at a steady speed. It is many times utilized in sports science and restoration settings to survey explicit muscle gatherings' solidarity and perseverance.

Muscle Lopsidedness Evaluation: Solid uneven characters, where certain muscles are more grounded or more vulnerable than their partners, can influence both day to day routine and sports execution. Appraisals can recognize these uneven characters and guide remedial activities.

Preparing for Solid Strength

Obstruction Preparing: The foundation of strong strength improvement is opposition preparing. This incorporates practices with free loads, machines, obstruction groups, or bodyweight opposition. Compound activities like squats, deadlifts, and seat presses are especially viable for developing generally speaking fortitude.

Moderate Over-burden: Persistently challenge the muscles by progressively expanding the obstruction or force of activities. This guideline of moderate over-burden invigorates muscle development and strength gains.

Appropriate Strategy: Keeping up with legitimate structure during opposition practices is fundamental to forestall injury and guarantee that the expected muscle bunches are actually focused on.

Variety: Incorporate various activities that target different muscle gatherings to forestall levels and advance adjusted improvement.

Rest and Recuperation: Muscles need satisfactory opportunity to recuperate and fix after difficult exercises. Overtraining can prompt weariness and frustrate strength gains.

Nourishment: Consume a decent eating routine wealthy in protein to help muscle development and fix. Legitimate hydration is likewise significant for execution and recuperation.

Consistency: Consistency is key in strength preparing. Ordinary exercises, preferably 2-4 times each week, are important to see huge upgrades.

Periodization: Integrate periodization into preparing plans, where force and volume are fluctuated over the long run to streamline gains and forestall abuse wounds.

Individualization: Designer preparing projects to individual objectives and requirements. Competitors in various games might require specific preparation regimens.

Recuperation Procedures: Use recuperation systems like extending, froth rolling, and back rub to lessen muscle irritation and improve adaptability.

1.3 Purpose of the Book

Books have been a basic piece of human civilization for quite a long time. They act as vaults of information, vehicles of narrating, and instruments for correspondence. Notwithstanding, the motivation behind a book can change essentially, incorporating many expectations and objectives. In this investigation, we will dig into the complex motivation behind a book, looking at its importance in training, diversion, data spread, social protection, and self-improvement.

1. **Schooling and Information Move**
1. **Reading material:** Instructive books intended for formal learning conditions, like schools and colleges, are instrumental in conferring information and abilities. They give an organized educational program, activities, and clarifications to work with the growing experience.
2. **Reference Books:** Reference books, word references, and instructional pamphlets act as supplies of data. They empower people to rapidly get to realities, definitions, and clarifications, making them significant instruments for exploration and critical thinking.
3. **Self improvement and Instructive Aides:** Books in this classification plan to teach perusers about unambiguous points or give direction to personal development. Models remember books for

language learning, individual budget, and profession improvement.

4. **Scholastic Exploration:** Scholarly and academic books are basic for the progression of information in different fields. These books present inside and out

research discoveries, hypotheses, and basic examinations, adding to the scholarly talk of society.

2. Diversion and Break

1. **Books:** Fictitious books transport perusers to fanciful settings, acquaint them with fascinating characters, and weave charming stories. Whether it's an outright exhilarating secret, an inspiring sentiment, or a fantastical experience, books offer a getaway from the real world.

2. **Brief tales:** Brief tale assortments give reduced down diversion, ideal for a fast redirection or a short reprieve from day to day existence. They frequently convey a succinct story with a punchy end.

3. **Verse:** Verse books offer a one of a kind type of imaginative articulation, utilizing language and symbolism to inspire feelings, contemplations, and tangible encounters. They can be both engaging and provocative.

4. **Realistic Books and Comics:** These books consolidate visual craftsmanship with narrating, making a dynamic and drawing in type of diversion. Realistic books and comics take care of a great many classes and crowds.

3. Data Scattering and News coverage

1. **True to life and Insightful News-casting:** Books in this class cover a tremendous range of subjects, from governmental issues and history to science and innovation. They intend to illuminate,

teach, and at times challenge winning convictions or uncover stowed away insights.

2. **Journals and Self-portrayals:** Individual accounts, diaries, and personal histories permit people to share their background, offering experiences into their one of a kind excursions and viewpoints.

3. **Assessment and Editorial:** Books that offer individual viewpoints, critique, and examination can shape public talk and impact social, political, and social conversations.

4. **News and Current Undertakings:** A few books are committed to reporting and dissecting recent developments, furnishing perusers with a more profound comprehension of contemporary issues.

4. Social Protection and Legacy

1. **Authentic Records:** Verifiable books describe previous occasions, times, and civic establishments. They assist with safeguarding verifiable information, offering bits of knowledge into the advancement of social orders, societies, and innovations.

2. **Old stories and Legends:** Books that incorporate fables, fantasies, and legends add to the conservation of social legacy. They keep up with the narrating customs and convictions of different networks.

3. **Recipe Books and Cookbooks:** Culinary books assume a part in protecting culinary customs, recipes, and cooking procedures extraordinary to various districts and societies.

4. **Craftsmanship and Engineering:** Books on workmanship and design report crafted by specialists, planners, and their inventive strategies, guaranteeing that their commitments to culture are recollected.

5. Self-improvement and Motivation

1. **Self improvement and Inspirational Books:** These books give procedures to self-awareness, building fearlessness, putting forth objectives, and defeating obstructions. They expect to enable perusers to lead additional satisfying lives.

2. **Accounts and Examples of overcoming adversity:** Learning about the lives and accomplishments of fruitful people can move others to seek after their fantasies and objectives.

3. **Philosophical and Otherworldly Works:** Books investigating reasoning, otherworldliness, and existential inquiries offer perusers a more profound comprehension of themselves and their general surroundings.

4. **Administration and The executives:** Books on authority, the board, and business offer significant bits of knowledge into successful initiative styles, hierarchical techniques, and dynamic cycles.

6. Social and Political Change

1. **Promotion and Activism:** Books composed by activists, supporters, and social reformers shed light on major problems and call for change. They can be instrumental in preparing general assessment.

2. **Political Compositions:** A few books, like political compositions and declarations, spread out political belief systems, standards, and dreams for a superior society.

3. **Basic liberties and Civil rights:** Books zeroing in on common freedoms, civil rights, and correspondence add to public mindfulness and conversations on these basic themes.

4. **Natural Worries:** Books on natural issues, protection, and manageability can bring issues to light about environmental difficulties and advance capable stewardship of the planet.

7. Individual Reflection and Articulation

1. **Journals and Diaries:** Individual journals and diaries act as confidential spaces for people to record their contemplations, encounters, and sentiments.
2. **Exploratory writing:** Experimental writing, including verse, papers, and individual stories, permits writers to offer their deepest viewpoints and feelings while interfacing with perusers on an individual level.
3. **Fiction as Investigation:** A writers use fiction to investigate complex subjects, feelings, and moral issues, welcoming perusers to consider the human condition.
4. **Workmanship and Photography Books:** These books grandstand visual craftsmanship and photography as types of individual articulation, conveying feelings, viewpoints, and style.

Chapter 2

Muscle Anatomy and Physiology

Muscles, the powerful motors of the human body, are the wonderful tissues answerable for empowering development, keeping up with stance, and carrying out fundamental roles. Understanding muscle life systems and physiology is vital to grasping the complexities of human development and the basic rules that oversee our capacity to lift, run, inhale, and even grin. In this exhaustive investigation, we set out on an excursion through the complicated universe of muscle tissue, from minute parts to the perceptible capabilities shape our day to day routines.

1. **Muscle Types**
1. **Skeletal Muscle**

   Skeletal muscles are the most unmistakable sort of muscle. They are answerable for deliberate developments, like strolling, running, and lifting loads. These muscles are connected to bones through ligaments and are under cognizant control. Skeletal muscles likewise assume a crucial part in keeping up with pose and creating intensity to control internal heat level.

2. Smooth Muscle

Smooth muscle is tracked down in the walls of interior organs, veins, and different body frameworks. Not at all like skeletal muscle, smooth muscle is compulsory, meaning it contracts without cognizant exertion. It controls capabilities like absorption, blood stream, and the development of substances through empty organs.

3. Heart Muscle

Cardiovascular muscle is elite to the heart and is liable for siphoning blood all through the body. It has a special capacity to contract musically and persistently without weariness. Like smooth muscle, heart muscle is additionally compulsory.

II. Life structures of Skeletal Muscle

1. Muscle Filaments

Muscle filaments, otherwise called muscle cells, are the structure blocks of skeletal muscles. These stretched cells contain numerous myofibrils, which are answerable for muscle constriction. Myofibrils, thus, comprise of rehashing units called sarcomeres. Sarcomeres are the practical units of muscle constriction and are made out of good and bad fibers.

2. Connective Tissues

Skeletal muscles are wrapped in layers of connective tissues that give construction and backing. The furthest layer, called the epimysium, encompasses the whole muscle. Inside the muscle, heaps of muscle filaments are gathered into fascicles, each encased by the perimysium. At last, individual muscle strands are ensheathed by the endomysium.

3. Ligaments

Ligaments are thick, stringy connective tissues that append muscles to bones. They communicate the power produced by muscle withdrawals to the skeleton, taking into account development. Ligaments are known for their surprising elasticity and assume a basic part in the biomechanics of development.

III. The Sliding Fiber Hypothesis

Muscle compression is a mind boggling process that happens at the sub-atomic level inside sarcomeres. The sliding fiber hypothesis is a central idea in muscle physiology that makes sense of how muscles contract. It includes the connection between two sorts of protein fibers: actin and myosin.

1. **Actin and Myosin**

   Actin and myosin are the essential proteins liable for muscle constriction. Actin fibers are flimsy and stretch out across the sarcomere, while myosin fibers are thicker and cross-over with actin. At the point when a muscle contracts, myosin makes a bee-line for actin and pull the meager fibers toward the focal point of the sarcomere.

2. **Cross-Extension Cycling**

The course of muscle constriction includes a rehashed pattern of cross-span development and separation. At the point when calcium particles are delivered inside the muscle cell, they tie to troponin, a protein that manages the place of tropomyosin on the actin fiber. This connection uncovered restricting locales on the actin fibers,

permitting myosin heads to join and turn, pulling the actin fibers toward the middle. The energy for this cycle comes from adenosine triphosphate (ATP).

IV. Brain Control of Muscle Withdrawal

The commencement and guideline of muscle compressions are heavily influenced by the sensory system. Muscles get signals from engine neurons that start in the cerebrum and spinal rope. This neuromuscular association guarantees exact control of muscle developments.

1. **Engine Units**
   Engine units are the utilitarian units of muscle control. Each engine unit comprises of an engine neuron and the muscle strands it innervates. Engine units fluctuate in size, with little engine units controlling fine developments and bigger engine units answerable for additional strong constrictions. The enrollment of engine units assumes a crucial part in directing the strength of muscle constrictions.

2. **Neuromuscular Intersection**
   The neuromuscular intersection is where the engine neuron meets the muscle fiber. At the point when an activity potential arrives at the finish of an engine neuron, it sets off the arrival of synapses, like acetylcholine, into the synaptic parted. Acetylcholine ties to receptors on the muscle fiber's film, prompting depolarization and the age of an activity potential in the muscle fiber.

3. **Muscle Fiber Excitation**

The activity likely goes along the muscle fiber's film (sarcolemma) and profound into the muscle fiber by means of invaginations called T-tubules. This sign eventually comes to the sarcoplasmic reticulum, a particular organization of layers that stores calcium particles. The arrival of calcium particles from the sarcoplasmic reticulum starts the constriction interaction by restricting to troponin on the actin fibers.

V. Muscle Fiber Types

Skeletal muscles contain various kinds of muscle filaments, each with unmistakable attributes fit to specific capabilities and requests. Understanding these fiber types is fundamental for competitors, as they impact execution and preparing systems.

1. **Type I (Slow-Jerk) Muscle Strands**
   Slow-jerk muscle strands are portrayed by their perseverance abilities. They contract generally leisurely and are profoundly

impervious to exhaustion. Type I filaments are rich in mitochondria, which empower effective high-impact energy creation. They are
basically enrolled for exercises like significant distance running and keeping up with pose.

2. **Type II (Quick Jerk) Muscle Strands**

1. **Type IIa (Quick Oxidative Glycolytic):** These strands contract rapidly, have a moderate protection from exhaustion, and depend on both high-impact and anaerobic energy creation. They are associated with exercises like running and moderate-weightlifting.

2. **Type IIx (Quick Glycolytic):** Type IIx strands contract quickly and have a low protection from weakness. They principally utilize anaerobic energy creation and are enrolled for short eruptions of extraordinary movement, for example, powerlifting and bouncing.

People have a novel proportion of slow-jerk to quick jerk muscle strands, which can impact their athletic presentation and preparing inclinations.

VI. Muscle Constriction and Energy Digestion

Muscle constrictions require a ceaseless stock of energy, especially as ATP. The energy for muscle constrictions is gotten from different metabolic pathways, contingent upon the term and power of the action.

1. **ATP and Creatine Phosphate**

The prompt wellspring of energy for muscle withdrawals is ATP put away inside the muscle strands. Nonetheless, ATP holds are restricted and immediately drained during extreme focus exercises. Creatine phosphate, another high-energy particle put away in muscles, can quickly recover ATP during short eruptions of action, like weightlifting or running.

2. **Anaerobic Glycolysis**

At the point when the interest for ATP surpasses the limit of creatine phosphate, muscles go to anaerobic glycolysis. This cycle separates glucose without the requirement for oxygen, creating ATP and lactate as results. Anaerobic glycolysis is essential for present moment, focused energy endeavors however prompts muscle weariness and the "consuming" sensation felt during exhausting activity.

3. **High-impact Breath**

For delayed exercises, for example, perseverance running or cycling, muscles depend on high-impact breath. This interaction utilizes oxygen to separate energy from glucose and unsaturated fats, delivering a lot bigger yield of ATP contrasted with anaerobic

pathways. Oxygen consuming breath permits muscles to support withdrawals for broadened periods without aggregating lactate.

VII. Muscle Development and Transformation

1. **Hypertrophy**
   Muscle hypertrophy alludes to the broadening of muscle filaments, basically determined by obstruction preparing. During opposition works out, microtears happen inside muscle filaments, provoking the body to fix and reconstruct them, prompting expanded fiber size and generally speaking muscle development. Hypertrophy can be accomplished through different preparation strategies, including moderate over-burden, which includes continuously expanding the opposition or burden over the long run.

2. **Hyperplasia**

Hyperplasia is the interaction by which new muscle filaments are framed, hypothetically expanding the complete number of muscle cells. While it has been seen in creature studies, hyperplasia in people stays a subject of discussion and progressing research.

VIII. Muscle Capability in Day to day existence

Past athletic pursuits, muscles assume a crucial part in ordinary exercises and by and large prosperity. They are associated with keeping up with act, working with development, and supporting indispensable capabilities like breath and dissemination.

1. **Postural Muscles**

   Postural muscles work persistently to keep an upstanding stance against the powers of gravity. These muscles are fundamental for dependability and equilibrium and are locked in while sitting, standing, or playing out any movement needing postural help.

2. **Respiratory Muscles**

   Muscles, for example, the stomach and intercostals are significant for relaxing. The stomach contracts and unwinds to make changes in thoracic volume, empowering inward breath and exhalation. Productive respiratory muscle capability is fundamental for keeping up with oxygen supply and eliminating carbon dioxide from the body.

3. **Heart Muscle Capability**

The cardiovascular muscle of the heart contracts musically to siphon blood all through the circulatory framework. This consistent, compulsory constriction is fundamental for keeping up with blood stream, conveying oxygen and supplements to tissues, and eliminating byproducts.

IX. Age-Related Changes and Muscle Wellbeing

Muscle wellbeing is basic all through the life expectancy, and age-related changes can affect muscle capability. Sarcopenia is the term used to depict the continuous loss of bulk and strength that happens with maturing. A few variables add to sarcopenia, including hormonal changes, decreased actual work, and modifications in protein digestion.

Neutralizing sarcopenia requires a complex methodology that incorporates customary opposition preparing, sufficient protein consumption, and keeping a functioning way of life. Thusly, people can protect bulk, strength, and practical autonomy as they age.

2.1 Muscle Types and Structure

Muscles are the powerful motors of the human body, driving development, keeping up with pose, and working with fundamental physiological capabilities. Understanding the complexities of muscle types and their hidden designs is pivotal for fathoming how our bodies move and capability. In this far reaching investigation of muscle types and construction, we will travel from the plainly visible grouping of muscles to the minute complexities of muscle filaments and the systems of muscle compression.

1. **Muscle Types**
1. **Skeletal Muscle**

   Skeletal muscles, frequently essentially alluded to as muscles, are the most natural and bountiful muscle type. They are joined to bones by means of ligaments and are answerable for deliberate developments, like strolling, running, and lifting objects. Skeletal muscles likewise assume a vital part in keeping up with act and creating intensity to direct internal heat level.

2. **Smooth Muscle**

   Smooth muscle is tracked down in the walls of interior organs, veins, and different body frameworks. Not at all like skeletal muscles, smooth muscles are compulsory, meaning they contract without cognizant control. They are answerable for fundamental capabilities, for example, absorption, guideline of blood stream, and the development of substances through empty organs.

3. **Cardiovascular Muscle**

Cardiovascular muscle is elite to the heart and assumes a focal part in siphoning blood all through the circulatory framework. It has an exceptional capacity to contract musically and constantly without exhaustion. Like smooth muscle, cardiovascular muscle is additionally compulsory and works independently affected by the heart's inward pacemaker.

II. Skeletal Muscle Design

Skeletal muscles, with their obvious appearance and essential job in willful development, act as the point of convergence for our investigation of muscle structure. To understand skeletal muscle completely, we should dig into its complex creation, from the tiny components of muscle strands to the perceptible association inside the body.

1. **Muscle Fiber (Muscle Cell)**

   Muscle strands, otherwise called muscle cells, are the principal building blocks of skeletal muscles. These extended, multinucleated cells run the length of the muscle and contain various myofibrils, the contractile components liable for muscle compression. Myofibrils, thusly, are made out of rehashing utilitarian units called sarcomeres.

2. **Sarcomere: The Contractile Unit**

   The sarcomere is the crucial practical unit of muscle withdrawal. It is the portion of a myofibril liable for creating power and shortening during muscle withdrawal. Sarcomeres comprise of two essential kinds of protein fibers: flimsy fibers (actin) and thick fibers (myosin). The cooperation between these fibers shapes the premise of muscle constriction.

3. **Connective Tissues**

Skeletal muscles are encompassed and interconnected by layers of connective tissues that offer primary help and coordination. Understanding these connective tissues is fundamental for getting a handle on how muscles capability as coordinated frameworks:

1. **Epimysium:** The furthest layer of connective tissue that encompasses the whole muscle.

2. **Perimysium:** Inside the muscle, heaps of muscle strands are assembled into fascicles, every one of which is encircled by the perimysium.
3. **Endomysium:** Individual muscle filaments inside a fascicle are wrapped by the endomysium.
4. **Ligaments:** Ligaments are thick, sinewy connective tissues that append muscles to bones. They act as the conductor for communicating the power produced by muscle

withdrawals to the skeleton, empowering development. Ligaments are known for their uncommon rigidity and are pivotal for the biomechanics of movement.

III. Sliding Fiber Hypothesis

1. **Actin and Myosin**
   Actin and myosin are the essential proteins answerable for muscle withdrawal. Actin fibers are meager and stretch out across the sarcomere, while myosin fibers are thicker and cross-over with actin. During muscle withdrawal, myosin makes a beeline for actin and pull the slim fibers toward the focal point of the sarcomere.
2. **Cross-Scaffold Cycling**

The course of muscle withdrawal involves a monotonous pattern of cross-span development and separation. At the point when calcium particles are delivered inside the muscle cell, they tie to troponin, an administrative protein liable for controlling the place of tropomyosin on the actin fiber. This association uncovered restricting destinations on the actin fibers, empowering myosin heads to connect and turn, consequently pulling the actin fibers toward the sarcomere's middle. The energy expected for this interaction is gotten from adenosine triphosphate (ATP).

IV. Brain Control of Muscle Withdrawal

The commencement and guideline of muscle withdrawals are coordinated by the sensory system, explicitly engine neurons. Understanding the brain control of muscle withdrawal is urgent for grasping how we order and direction developments.

1. **Engine Units**

   Engine units are the essential practical units of muscle control. Each engine unit includes an engine neuron and the muscle strands it innervates. Engine units fluctuate in size, with more modest engine units controlling fine, exact developments and bigger engine units liable for creating more powerful constrictions. The enrollment of engine units assumes a crucial part in managing the strength of muscle withdrawals.

2. **Neuromuscular Intersection**

   The neuromuscular intersection is the resource where an engine neuron speaks with a muscle fiber. At the point when an activity potential arrives at the engine neuron's end, it sets off the arrival of synapses, like acetylcholine, into the synaptic separated. Acetylcholine ties to receptors on the muscle fiber's film, starting depolarization and the ensuing age of an activity potential inside the muscle fiber.

3. **Muscle Fiber Excitation**

The activity potential proliferates along the muscle fiber's film, or sarcolemma, and profound into the fiber by means of specific invaginations known as T-tubules. Eventually, this sign reaches the sarcoplasmic reticulum, a complicated organization of layers that stores calcium particles. The arrival of calcium particles from the sarcoplasmic reticulum is the trigger for muscle compression, as they tie to troponin on the actin fibers.

V. Muscle Fiber Types

Skeletal muscles are made out of various sorts of muscle filaments, each described by remarkable properties and capabilities.

Understanding these muscle fiber types is fundamental for competitors and people intending to enhance their actual exhibition and preparing methodologies.

1. **Type I (Slow-Jerk) Muscle Filaments**
   Type I muscle filaments, frequently alluded to as sluggish jerk strands, are described by their perseverance abilities. These filaments contract generally leisurely and are exceptionally impervious to weariness. Type I strands are rich in mitochondria, which empower proficient vigorous energy creation. They are fundamentally selected for exercises requiring perseverance, like significant distance running and keeping up with act.
2. **Type II (Quick Jerk) Muscle Filaments**
1. **Type IIa (Quick Oxidative Glycolytic):** These filaments contract rapidly, have moderate weakness obstruction, and depend on both vigorous and anaerobic energy creation. They are engaged with exercises, for example, running and moderate-weight training.
2. **Type IIx (Quick Glycolytic):** Type IIx filaments contract quickly and have low weariness opposition. They essentially use anaerobic energy creation and are enrolled for short explosions of serious movement, for example, powerlifting and bouncing.

A singular's novel proportion of slow-jerk to quick jerk muscle strands can impact their athletic presentation and preparing inclinations.

VI. Muscle Compression and Energy Digestion

Muscle compressions request a persistent stockpile of energy, essentially as adenosine triphosphate (ATP). The wellspring of energy for muscle constrictions changes relying upon the span and power of the action.

1. **ATP and Creatine Phosphate**
   ATP is the prompt energy hotspot for muscle withdrawals. In any case, ATP holds are restricted and immediately drained during extreme focus exercises. Creatine phosphate, another high-energy atom put away in muscles, can quickly recover ATP during short eruptions of action, like weightlifting or running.
2. **Anaerobic Glycolysis**
   At the point when the interest for ATP surpasses the limit of creatine phosphate, muscles go to anaerobic glycolysis. This cycle separates glucose without the requirement for oxygen, creating ATP and lactate as side-effects. Anaerobic glycolysis is fundamental for present moment, extreme focus endeavors however prompts muscle weakness and the impression of "consuming" during exhausting activity.
3. **Vigorous Breath**

Drawn out exercises, for example, perseverance running or cycling, depend on high-impact breath. This interaction utilizes oxygen to extricate energy from glucose and unsaturated fats, creating a lot bigger yield of ATP contrasted with anaerobic pathways. High-impact breath permits muscles to support constrictions for broadened periods without aggregating lactate.

VII. Muscle Development and Transformation

1. **Hypertrophy**
   Muscle hypertrophy alludes to the development of muscle strands and is fundamentally instigated by obstruction preparing. During opposition works out, microtears happen inside muscle filaments, inciting the body to fix and modify them. This cycle brings about expanded fiber size and generally muscle development. Hypertrophy can be accomplished through different preparation methods, including moderate over-burden, which includes slowly expanding opposition or burden after some time.

2. Hyperplasia

Hyperplasia is the interaction by which new muscle strands are shaped, hypothetically expanding the complete number of muscle cells. While it has been seen in creature studies, hyperplasia in people stays a subject of discussion and progressing research.

VIII. Muscle Capability in Day to day existence

Muscles are basic for everyday exercises and generally prosperity, reaching out past athletic pursuits. They are instrumental in keeping up with pose, working with development, and supporting basic capabilities like breath and course.

1. **Postural Muscles**
   Postural muscles work consistently to support an upstanding stance against the powers of gravity. These muscles are essential for security and equilibrium and are locked in while sitting, standing, or playing out any movement needing postural help.

2. **Respiratory Muscles**
   Muscles, for example, the stomach and intercostals assume a crucial part in relaxing. The stomach contracts and unwinds, creating changes in thoracic volume that empower inward breath and exhalation. Effective respiratory muscle capability is fundamental for keeping up with oxygen supply and wiping out carbon dioxide from the body.

3. **Heart Muscle Capability**

The cardiovascular muscle of the heart contracts musically to siphon blood all through the circulatory framework. This steady, compulsory constriction is crucial for keeping up with blood stream, conveying oxygen and supplements to tissues, and eliminating side-effects.

IX. Age-Related Changes and Muscle Wellbeing

Muscle wellbeing is basic all through the life expectancy, and age-related changes can influence muscle capability. Sarcopenia, the steady loss of bulk and strength that happens with maturing, is a remarkable concern. A few elements add to sarcopenia, including hormonal changes, decreased actual work, and modifications in protein digestion.

Checking sarcopenia requires a complex methodology that incorporates ordinary opposition preparing, sufficient protein consumption, and keeping a functioning way of life. Thusly, people can protect bulk, strength, and practical autonomy as they age.

2.2 Neuromuscular Connection

The neuromuscular association, a wonder of natural designing, is a key cycle that permits us to perform even the easiest of developments and the most intricate of athletic accomplishments. This mind boggling interaction between the sensory system and solid framework shapes the premise of human movement and is a subject of tremendous interest and examination inside the areas of neuroscience, physiology, and sports science. In this complete investigation, we will dig into the neuromuscular association, revealing its components, its job in daily existence and sports execution, and the expected ramifications for recovery and execution upgrade.

Life systems and Physiology of the Neuromuscular Association

The neuromuscular association principally includes two primary parts: the sensory system and the strong framework. To comprehend this association, it is essential to look at the life structures and physiology of these frameworks and how they collaborate.

1.1 The Sensory system

The sensory system fills in as the director in the ensemble of development. It comprises of two primary parts: the focal sensory system (CNS) and the fringe sensory system (PNS).

The CNS, contained the mind and spinal line, assumes a focal part in organizing and handling data. At the point when we choose to play out a development, for example, lifting a glass of water, the mind conveys messages through the spinal rope to the fitting muscles to execute the activity.

1.2 The Fringe Sensory system

The PNS is a huge organization of nerves that stretch out from the spinal rope to each side of the body, including the muscles. It is through the PNS that the CNS speaks with muscles. The PNS can be additionally isolated into the physical and autonomic sensory systems. For our motivations, the substantial sensory system is of essential interest as it administers deliberate muscle development.

1.3 Neuromuscular Intersection

At the center of the neuromuscular association lies the neuromuscular intersection (NMJ), a specific neurotransmitter where nerves meet muscle strands. This intersection is the mark of correspondence between the sensory system and muscles. At the point when a sign from the CNS arrives at the NMJ, it sets off a progression of occasions that at last lead to muscle constriction.

The Course of Neuromuscular Transmission

2.1 Age of Nerve Motivation

Everything starts with the age of a nerve motivation in the CNS. At the point when you choose to play out an activity, for example, getting a pencil, the cerebrum conveys an electrical message down the spinal line to the engine neurons answerable for the muscles engaged with that activity.

2.2 Transmission Across the Neurotransmitter

After arriving at the neuromuscular intersection, the nerve drive should cross the synaptic split, a little hole between the sensitive spot and the muscle fiber. To navigate \

this hole, the nerve discharges synapses, fundamentally acetylcholine, which tie to receptors on the muscle fiber layer, known as the sarcolemma.

2.3 Muscle Fiber Excitation

The limiting of acetylcholine to receptors on the sarcolemma sets off an electrical motivation that movements along the muscle fiber's surface. This motivation enters profound into the muscle fiber by means of an organization of tubules known as the T-tubules.

2.4 Calcium Delivery

The T-tubules speak with the sarcoplasmic reticulum, a particular organelle inside muscle strands. This connection prompts the arrival of calcium particles into the muscle fiber's cytoplasm.

2.5 Muscle Compression

The presence of calcium particles in the muscle fiber starts a progression of compound responses that at last lead to muscle constriction. The contractile proteins actin and myosin associate, making the muscle fiber abbreviate, prompting muscle withdrawal. This constriction creates the power important to play out the ideal development.

2.6 End of Sign

When the nerve motivation has been sent and the muscle has gotten, the sign should be ended to consider unwinding. This cycle includes the breakdown of acetylcholine and the reuptake of calcium particles by the sarcoplasmic reticulum, returning the muscle to its resting state.

Significance of the Neuromuscular Association

Understanding the meaning of the neuromuscular association is significant in valuing its job in regular daily existence and sports execution.

3.1 Ordinary Developments

Each activity, from composing on a console to lifting a spoon, depends on the neuromuscular association. This complicated cycle guarantees that our developments are exact, controlled, and versatile to different assignments. Without this association, even the least complex activities would be unimaginable.

3.2 Games Execution

In the domain of sports and games, the neuromuscular association takes on added significance. Competitors should not exclusively have the option to execute exact developments yet additionally do as such with power and speed. The capacity to adjust the neuromuscular association through preparing and practice is fundamental for accomplishing maximized execution.

3.3 Restoration and Recuperation

At the point when wounds or neuromuscular problems disturb the association, restoration becomes fundamental. Non-intrusive treatment and designated practices expect to reestablish legitimate neuromuscular capability. Understanding the mechanics of this association is basic for planning viable recovery programs.

Elements Affecting Neuromuscular Capability

A few elements can impact the proficiency and viability of the neuromuscular association, both emphatically and adversely.

4.1 Age

Age essentially affects neuromuscular capability. As we age, the quantity of engine neurons and muscle strands diminishes, prompting a decrease in bulk and strength. This age-related decline can influence regular developments and athletic execution.

4.2 Preparation and Molding

Actual preparation and molding assume a critical part in improving the neuromuscular association. Explicit activities and preparing regimens can upgrade engine unit enlistment, coordination, and muscle fiber enrollment. Competitors and wellness devotees constantly look for ways of fining tune this association with succeed in their picked disciplines.

4.3 Sustenance

Sustenance is another significant element that can impact neuromuscular capability. Appropriate admission of fundamental supplements, for example, protein and minerals like calcium and magnesium, is indispensable for muscle withdrawal and nerve motivation transmission.

4.4 Neuromuscular Problems

Neuromuscular problems, for example, solid dystrophy or myasthenia gravis, can upset the neuromuscular association. These circumstances bring about muscle shortcoming,

exhaustion, and debilitated engine capability. The board and treatment frequently include resolving the hidden neurological and solid issues.

Upgrading Neuromuscular Capability

5.1 Strength Preparing

Strength preparing is a foundation of neuromuscular improvement. It includes practices that challenge muscles and the neuromuscular association, prompting expanded bulk, strength, and coordination. Procedures like obstruction preparing, plyometrics, and isometric activities target various parts of neuromuscular turn of events.

5.2 Plyometrics and Hazardous Preparation

For competitors hoping to amplify power and hazardousness, plyometric practices are fundamental. These developments, which include fast muscle extending and shortening, assist with upgrading the stretch reflex and improve the neuromuscular association's capacity to rapidly create force.

5.3 Neurofeedback and Biofeedback

State of the art advances like neurofeedback and biofeedback give constant data about neuromuscular capability. Competitors and people can utilize this criticism to refine their coordinated abilities, concentration, and unwinding, at last prompting worked on neuromuscular execution.

5.4 Brain Body Procedures

Mind-body strategies, like yoga and kendo, center around the incorporation of mental and actual parts of development. These practices can upgrade neuromuscular control, equilibrium, and coordination.

5.5 Nourishment and Enhancements

Nourishing methodologies and enhancements can uphold neuromuscular capability. Legitimate hydration, adjusted sustenance, and enhancements like creatine and stretched chain amino acids can support muscle recuperation and execution.

Clinical Applications and Future Bearings

The comprehension of the neuromuscular association has extensive ramifications in different fields, including medical services, sports science, and innovation.

6.1 Clinical Applications

In medical services, the investigation of the neuromuscular association is instrumental in diagnosing and treating neuromuscular problems. Treatments and intercessions pointed toward streamlining this association are constantly developing, offering desire to people with conditions that influence their engine capability.

6.2 Games Science

In the domain of sports science, progressing examination into the neuromuscular association illuminates preparing strategies, injury counteraction methodologies, and execution upgrade procedures. As our comprehension extends, competitors are probably going to accomplish much more noteworthy impressive performances, speed, and accuracy.

6.3 Innovation and Neuromuscular Points of interaction

Propels in innovation are additionally ready to reform the field. Neuromuscular connection points, which permit direct correspondence between the sensory system and outer gadgets, hold the possibility to reestablish capability to people with loss of motion and improve human-machine communications.

6.4 Moral Contemplations

As we investigate the outskirts of neuromuscular science and innovation, moral contemplations become principal. Inquiries concerning the utilization of neuromuscular upgrades, security, and the potential for abuse should be painstakingly inspected.

Chapter 3

Muscle Contraction and Energy Systems

Muscle compression is a crucial physiological cycle that empowers human development and capability. Whether it's lifting a weighty item, running a long distance race, or just squinting our eyes, muscle withdrawal is at the core, all things considered, To support these exercises, our bodies depend on a perplexing interaction of energy frameworks. In this thorough investigation, we will dig into the mechanics of muscle constriction and the different energy frameworks that power our developments, revealing insight into the mind boggling physiological cycles that underlie our capacity to move.

Muscle Compression

Muscle compression is the cycle by which muscle filaments produce force and abbreviate long. This fundamental capability is liable for all deliberate and compulsory developments in the human body.

1.1 Life structures of Muscle Tissue

Skeletal Muscle: Skeletal muscles are the most well-known type and are joined to bones by ligaments. They are answerable for willful developments, like strolling and lifting loads.

Smooth Muscle: Smooth muscles are tracked down in the walls of organs, veins, and the gastrointestinal system. They are answerable for compulsory developments like peristalsis and keeping up with organ tone.

Cardiovascular Muscle: Heart muscle makes up the heart and is liable for the cadenced constrictions that siphon blood all through the body.

1.2 Instrument of Muscle Withdrawal

1.2.1 Excitation-Constriction Coupling

Excitation-compression coupling is the cycle by which a muscle fiber is invigorated to contract. It includes the accompanying advances:

Nerve motivations travel from the cerebrum or spinal line to the muscle strands by means of engine neurons.

The nerve motivation arrives at the neuromuscular intersection, where it sets off the arrival of the synapse acetylcholine.

Acetylcholine ties to receptors on the muscle fiber's layer, known as the sarcolemma, prompting the age of an electrical motivation that spreads along the muscle fiber.

1.2.2 Sliding Fiber Hypothesis

The sliding fiber hypothesis makes sense of how muscle withdrawal happens at the sub-atomic level. It includes the collaboration between two key proteins: actin and myosin.

At the point when a muscle fiber gets an electrical drive, it sets calcium particles free from its sarcoplasmic reticulum.

These calcium particles tie to a protein called troponin, which permits myosin heads to connect to actin fibers.

Myosin heads then turn, pulling the actin fibers towards the focal point of the sarcomere (the contractile unit of a muscle fiber).

This sliding of actin and myosin fibers abbreviates the sarcomere, prompting muscle withdrawal.

1.2.3 Cross-Scaffold Cycling

Cross-span cycling is the dreary connection, turning, and separation of myosin heads to actin fibers. This interaction go on as long as calcium particles and ATP (adenosine triphosphate) are accessible.

1.2.4 Unwinding

Muscle unwinding happens when the nerve motivation stops, and calcium particles are effectively moved once again into the sarcoplasmic reticulum. This interaction permits the actin and myosin fibers to slide separated, extending the muscle fiber and making it unwind.

1.3 Sorts of Muscle Withdrawal

1.3.1 Isometric Compression

In isometric compressions, the muscle produces force without changing its length. For instance, when you hold a weighty article without lifting it, your muscles are participated in an isometric constriction. Isometric withdrawals assume a vital part in balancing out joints and keeping up with act.

1.3.2 Isotonic Compression

Concentric Constriction: In concentric compressions, the muscle abbreviates as it produces force. For instance, when you play out a bicep twist and lift a free weight, your biceps go through concentric constrictions.

Unusual Withdrawal: Flighty constrictions happen when a muscle protracts while producing force. For example, when you bring down a load during a bicep twist, your biceps are going through unusual withdrawals. Unusual withdrawals are fundamental for controlling the drop of a weight and decelerating body developments.

1.3.3 Muscle Jerk

Idle Stage: The concise period between the nerve motivation and the beginning of muscle constriction.

Compression Stage: The stage during which the muscle creates pressure and abbreviates.

Unwinding Stage: The period when the muscle gets back to its resting length.

Energy Frameworks for Muscle Constriction

To control muscle compression, our bodies depend on different energy frameworks that give the fundamental fuel to muscle cells to work. These energy frameworks work all the while and are called after relying upon the power and length of actual work.

2.1 ATP: The General Energy Cash

Adenosine triphosphate (ATP) is frequently alluded to as the "general energy cash" of cells since it stores and moves energy inside the cell. ATP is basic for muscle constriction since it gives the quick energy expected to cross-span cycling and myosin-actin collaborations.

2.2 Phosphagen Framework (ATP-CP Framework)

The phosphagen framework is the prompt wellspring of ATP for short explosions of extreme focus action, normally going on for around 10 seconds. It principally depends on the transformation of creatine phosphate (CP) into ATP in a response catalyzed by the catalyst creatine kinase.

Creatine Kinase: Creatine kinase catalyzes the exchange of a phosphate bunch from CP to ADP (adenosine diphosphate), framing ATP.

This framework is fundamental for exercises, for example, running, bouncing, and lifting significant burdens, where fast and strong muscle withdrawals are required.

2.3 Anaerobic Glycolytic Framework (Glycolysis)

The anaerobic glycolytic framework is answerable for giving energy during extreme focus exercises enduring from around 30 seconds to 2 minutes. It fundamentally depends on glucose, either from blood glucose or put away glycogen inside muscle cells.

Glycolysis: Glycolysis is a progression of compound responses that separate glucose into pyruvate, producing a limited quantity of ATP simultaneously.

Since glycolysis doesn't need oxygen, it is viewed as an anaerobic energy framework. Be that as it may, it produces lactic corrosive as a side-effect, prompting muscle exhaustion and touchiness when it gathers.

2.4 High-impact Framework (Oxidative Phosphorylation)

The high-impact framework is the essential energy hotspot for supported, low-to-direct power exercises enduring over 2 minutes. It depends on the oxidation of starches, fats, and, less significantly, proteins to deliver ATP. The essential pathway for high-impact ATP creation is oxidative phosphorylation, which happens inside the mitochondria of muscle cells.

Oxidative Phosphorylation: This cycle includes the electron transport chain and the creation of ATP from the breakdown of glucose and unsaturated fats within the sight of oxygen.

The vigorous framework is profoundly effective at producing ATP however works more leisurely than the anaerobic frameworks. It is the predominant energy framework during exercises like running, cycling, and perseverance occasions.

2.5 Interchange of Energy Frameworks

As a general rule, every one of the three energy frameworks (phosphagen, anaerobic glycolytic, and oxygen consuming) work all the while to differing degrees during actual work. The decision of energy framework relies upon elements like activity force, term, and the accessibility of oxygen.

Beginning Energy Commitment: The phosphagen framework gives quick ATP to the initial couple of moments of action.

Shift to Anaerobic Glycolytic: As action proceeds, the anaerobic glycolytic framework turns out to be progressively significant for providing ATP.

Vigorous Strength: For longer-span exercises, the high-impact framework turns into the predominant wellspring of ATP, and it keeps on giving energy for however long oxygen is accessible.

Elements Impacting Energy Framework Use

The usage of various energy frameworks during actual work is impacted by a few elements, including hereditary qualities, preparing, and nourishment.

3.1 Hereditary Variables

People might have hereditary inclinations that make them more fit to particular sorts of proactive tasks. For instance, certain individuals might succeed in powerlifting because of a characteristic penchant for speedy energy framework usage, while others might succeed in high-intensity games because of an effective vigorous framework.

3.2 Preparation Transformations

Further developed ATP-CP Framework: Opposition preparing and intense cardio exercise (HIIT) can improve the limit of the ATP-CP framework, considering more unstable power.

Upgraded Anaerobic Glycolytic Framework: Span preparing and sport-explicit drills can work on the anaerobic glycolytic framework's capacity to create ATP without collecting unnecessary lactic corrosive.

Vigorous Perseverance: Long-term, low-to-direct power preparing, for example, distance running or cycling, can upgrade the high-impact framework's ability for ATP creation and oxygen usage.

3.3 Nourishment

Starches: Sugars are the body's favored energy source, particularly during extreme focus work out. Consuming carbs previously and during activity can assist with supporting execution.

Fats: Fats give a huge wellspring of energy during lower-power, longer-term exercises. Perseverance competitors frequently depend on put away fat for fuel.

Proteins: While not an essential energy source, proteins can add to ATP creation, particularly during delayed practice when other fuel sources are exhausted.

3.4 Oxygen Accessibility

The accessibility of oxygen significantly impacts energy framework usage. Exercises acted in an oxygen-rich climate, like running or swimming, principally depend on the high-impact framework. On the other hand, exercises that request quick energy creation in an oxygen-exhausted state, such as running, vigorously connect with the anaerobic frameworks.

Useful Applications and Execution Advancement

Understanding muscle compression and energy frameworks has commonsense applications for competitors, wellness lovers, and anybody trying to advance their actual execution.

4.1 Preparation Program Plan

Extreme cardio exercise (HIIT): HIIT substitutes short explosions of focused energy practice with brief recuperation periods, really testing both the ATP-CP and anaerobic glycolytic frameworks.

Aerobic exercise: Perseverance competitors participate in longer, lower-power instructional courses to improve the vigorous framework's ability.

4.2 Healthful Systems

Starch Stacking: Carb stacking can assist with expanding glycogen stores before perseverance occasions.

Protein Admission: Sufficient protein consumption upholds muscle fix and can add to ATP creation during delayed work out.

Hydration: Keeping up with legitimate hydration is pivotal for energy framework capability and generally speaking execution.

4.3 Recuperation Strategies

Compelling recuperation methodologies assist competitors with returning from extreme preparation and contest. Methods like extending, knead, and cryotherapy can lessen muscle irritation and backing muscle recuperation, considering better energy framework usage in ensuing meetings.

4.4 Checking and Following

Progresses in innovation have furnished competitors with apparatuses to screen and track energy framework usage progressively. Wearable wellness trackers, pulse screens, and physiological testing permit people to assemble information that can direct preparation and streamline execution.

Clinical Ramifications and Future Bearings

The comprehension of muscle constriction and energy frameworks has significant clinical ramifications and opens up roads for future exploration.

5.1 Clinical Ramifications

Restoration: Information on energy frameworks is imperative in planning recovery programs for people recuperating from wounds.

Actual advisors tailor activities to modify muscle strength and capability while limiting the gamble of re-injury.

Solid Problems: Understanding muscle constriction is essential for diagnosing and treating strong problems, for example, strong dystrophy and myasthenia gravis.

Forestalling Muscle Weariness: In clinical settings, overseeing muscle exhaustion is fundamental for patients with persistent circumstances or neuromuscular problems. Strategies to limit muscle exhaustion can work on generally speaking personal satisfaction.

5.2 Future Headings

Biomechanics and Mechanical technology: Investigation into muscle constriction mechanics educates the plan regarding biomechanical gadgets and automated frameworks that copy human development. These developments have applications in medical care, prosthetics, and actual recovery.

Hereditary Mediations: Progressions in hereditary exploration might prompt intercessions that improve energy framework proficiency or moderate muscle-related messes.

Advancing Execution: As how we might interpret energy frameworks develops, we can expect more exact preparation and wholesome techniques that improve execution and lessen the gamble of injury.

3.1 Muscle Contraction Mechanisms

Muscle withdrawal is a wonderful physiological cycle that empowers the human body to play out a huge range of developments, from the straightforward demonstration of getting a pencil to the intricate complexities of athletic execution. At the center of this unique cycle lie many-sided sub-atomic components that arrange the compression of muscle strands. In this extensive investigation, we will dig into the entrancing universe of muscle constriction components, unwinding the atomic occasions that underlie our capacity to move.

Life systems and Physiology of Skeletal Muscle

Before we dig into the systems of muscle withdrawal, understanding the life structures and physiology of skeletal muscle, the kind of muscle answerable for willful movements is significant.

1.1 Skeletal Muscle Construction

Skeletal muscles are made out of various muscle strands packaged together. These muscle strands are long, round and hollow cells that can traverse the whole length of the muscle. They are encased in connective tissue sheaths and are lavishly vascularized and innervated.

1.2 Sarcomeres: The Practical Units of Muscle

Actin Fibers: Flimsy fibers made out of the protein actin.

Myosin Fibers: Thick fibers made out of the protein myosin.

The plan of actin and myosin fibers inside the sarcomere is vital to grasping muscle constriction.

The Sliding Fiber Hypothesis

The sliding fiber hypothesis is the predominant model that makes sense of how muscle constriction happens at the sub-atomic level. This hypothesis recommends that muscle strands contract when the actin fibers slide past the myosin fibers, bringing about the shortening of the sarcomere and, thusly, the muscle fiber.

2.1 Sub-atomic Parts

Actin: Actin is a globular protein that structures long chains and is the meager fibers of the sarcomere.

Myosin: Myosin is an engine protein with a novel construction, including a head locale that contains ATPase movement.

Troponin and Tropomyosin: These administrative proteins are related with actin fibers and assume a vital part in muscle compression.

2.2 Strides of Muscle Withdrawal

2.2.1 Resting State

In the resting state, myosin heads are positioned and prepared to associate with actin. Nonetheless, this collaboration is forestalled by the presence of tropomyosin, which covers the myosin-restricting locales on actin.

2.2.2 Calcium Delivery

At the point when a nerve motivation arrives at the neuromuscular intersection, it sets off the arrival of calcium particles (Ca2+) from the sarcoplasmic reticulum, a specific organelle inside the muscle fiber.

2.2.3 Cross-Scaffold Development

The delivered calcium particles tie to troponin, causing a conformational change that moves tropomyosin away from the myosin-restricting destinations on actin. This permits myosin heads to tie to actin, framing cross-spans.

2.2.4 Power Stroke

When cross-spans are shaped, myosin heads turn, pulling the actin fibers toward the focal point of the sarcomere. This is alluded to as the power stroke.

2.2.5 ATP Hydrolysis and Cross-Extension Separation

After the power stroke, myosin heads discharge ADP and inorganic phosphate (Pi), and ATP ties to them. This limiting makes myosin confine from actin.

2.2.6 Resetting the Cross-Extension

ATP is then hydrolyzed to ADP and Pi, giving energy to the myosin head to get back to its positioned position. The cross-span is currently reset and prepared for one more pattern of connection and separation.

2.2.7 Rehashed Cycles

These means are rehashed quickly the length of calcium particles are available, ATP is accessible, and nerve motivations keep on invigorating the muscle fiber. This dull pattern of cross-span arrangement and separation brings about the shortening of the sarcomere, prompting muscle constriction.

Neuromuscular Intersection and Sign Transmission

Muscle constriction is started by nerve driving forces that begin in the focal sensory system and travel to the neuromuscular intersection, where they animate the arrival of synapses. Understanding this sign transmission is fundamental to grasp how muscle constriction is controlled.

3.1 Neuromuscular Intersection (NMJ)

The neuromuscular intersection is the neurotransmitter or association point between an engine neuron and a muscle fiber. It is where the nerve signal is communicated to the muscle, prompting withdrawal.

3.2 Sign Transmission Steps

3.2.1 Nerve Motivation

A nerve motivation, or activity potential, goes down an engine neuron from the focal sensory system to the neuromuscular intersection.

3.2.2 Synapse Delivery

At the point when the nerve drive arrives at the finish of the engine neuron, it sets off the arrival of the synapse acetylcholine (ACh) from vesicles in the neuron's synaptic end bulbs.

3.2.3 ACh Restricting

ACh diffuses across the synaptic separated and ties to receptors on the sarcolemma (muscle fiber layer).

3.2.4 Muscle Fiber Excitation

The limiting of ACh to its receptors on the sarcolemma prompts an adjustment of the electrical charge of the muscle fiber. This change, called the end-plate potential, starts the proliferation of an activity likely along the sarcolemma and into the T-tubules.

3.2.5 Calcium Delivery

The activity possible going down the T-tubules causes the sarcoplasmic reticulum to deliver calcium particles (Ca2+) into the cytoplasm of the muscle fiber.

3.2.6 Muscle Withdrawal (Cross-Scaffold Cycling)

As depicted before, the presence of calcium particles starts the cross-span cycling among actin and myosin, prompting muscle withdrawal.

Guideline of Muscle Withdrawal

The exact guideline of muscle withdrawal is fundamental to guarantee that muscles possibly contract when and to the degree important. The administrative proteins troponin and tropomyosin assume a focal part in this cycle.

4.1 Troponin and Tropomyosin Complex

Inside the sarcomere, troponin and tropomyosin cooperate to control muscle withdrawal. Troponin is a complex of three subunits: troponin C, troponin I, and troponin T.

4.2 Job of Troponin and Tropomyosin

Tropomyosin lies along the actin fibers and covers the myosin-restricting destinations on actin in the resting state. Troponin, when bound to calcium particles, goes through a conformational change that moves tropomyosin away from the myosin-restricting destinations, permitting cross-span development and muscle constriction to happen.

4.3 Calcium Guideline

The centralization of calcium particles in the cytoplasm is a basic controller of muscle constriction. At the point when calcium particles are low, tropomyosin forestalls the cooperation among actin and myosin. Notwithstanding, when calcium particles are delivered, as depicted in the neuromuscular intersection segment, troponin ties to them and triggers the development of tropomyosin, empowering muscle compression.

Kinds of Muscle Constriction

Muscle withdrawals can be characterized into different sorts in light of the idea of the development and the control of the sensory system.

5.1 Isometric Constriction

Isometric constrictions happen when muscle filaments create force without changing their length. These compressions are fundamental for keeping up with act and settling joints. For instance, when you hold a weighty item without lifting or bringing down it, your muscles participate in an isometric withdrawal.

5.2 Isotonic Withdrawal

Concentric Constriction: In concentric withdrawals, the muscle abbreviates as it produces force. For instance, during the vertical period of a bicep twist, your biceps go through concentric compressions.

Flighty Compression: Unpredictable constrictions happen when a muscle protracts while creating force. For example, during the descending period of a bicep twist, your biceps are going through flighty compressions. Flighty compressions are critical for controlling the plunge of a weight and decelerating body developments.

5.3 Muscle Jerk

Inert Stage: The short time frame between the nerve motivation and the beginning of muscle constriction.

Compression Stage: The stage during which the muscle creates strain and abbreviates.

Unwinding Stage: The period when the muscle gets back to its resting length.

Variables Affecting Muscle Withdrawal

A few elements impact muscle withdrawal, including brain input, muscle fiber type, and engine unit enrollment.

6.1 Brain Information

The sensory system assumes a focal part in managing muscle withdrawal. The recurrence and strength of brain motivations shipped off muscle strands decide the power and term of constriction. Engine neurons control the initiation of muscle filaments through engine unit enlistment.

6.2 Muscle Fiber Type

Type I (Slow-Jerk) Muscle Strands: These filaments are adjusted for perseverance and are rich in mitochondria and myoglobin, giving them a red appearance. They are appropriate for exercises like significant distance running.

Type II (Quick Jerk) Muscle Strands: Type II filaments are additionally partitioned into

Type IIa and Type IIb (or IIx) strands. Type IIa filaments have moderate perseverance and strength qualities, while Type IIb strands are upgraded for short eruptions of extreme focus movement however weariness rapidly. Runners commonly have a higher extent of Type II strands.

The creation of muscle fiber types in a singular's muscles can impact their athletic presentation and muscle contractile capacities.

6.3 Engine Unit Enrollment

Engine units comprise of an engine neuron and all the muscle strands it innervates. The enrollment of engine units by the sensory system decides the power created during muscle compression. More modest, low-limit engine units are enrolled first for low-power exercises, while bigger, high-edge engine units are enlisted as the interest for force increments.

Clinical Ramifications and Exploration Headings

Understanding muscle withdrawal systems has huge clinical ramifications in the fields of restoration, sports medication, and the treatment of neuromuscular issues.

7.1 Restoration

Information on muscle compression systems guides actual advisors in planning compelling restoration programs for people recuperating from wounds or medical procedures. Custom-made practices assist with remaking muscle strength and capability, frequently utilizing standards, for example, moderate obstruction preparing.

7.2 Games Medication

In sports medication, a comprehension of muscle constriction systems is fundamental for diagnosing and treating muscle wounds, spasms, and weariness. It additionally advises the plan regarding preparing regimens pointed toward upgrading athletic execution and forestalling wounds.

7.3 Neuromuscular Issues

Muscle compression components are key to the finding and treatment of neuromuscular issues, for example, strong dystrophy, myasthenia gravis, and amyotrophic horizontal sclerosis (ALS). Research in this space investigates expected treatments to reestablish or upgrade muscle capability in people with these circumstances.

7.4 Future Exploration Bearings

Biomechanics: Progressions in biomechanics research plan to work on how we might interpret muscle mechanics and productivity.

Neuromuscular Connection points: Arising advancements like neuromuscular points of interaction hold the commitment of reestablishing development in people with loss of motion.

Hereditary Intercessions: Investigation into hereditary mediations might offer better approaches to improve muscle capability and treat muscle-related messes.

3.2 Energy Systems in Muscle Function

The capacity to move is a principal quality of living creatures, and it is especially articulated in the animals of the world collectively. Muscles assume a focal part in working with development, and to do as such, they require a constant stock of energy. This energy is gotten from different energy frameworks inside the body, each custom-made to satisfy the particular needs of various exercises. In this thorough investigation, we will dive into the captivating universe of energy frameworks in muscle capability, disentangling the mind boggling processes that power our capacity to move and perform proactive tasks.

The Lively Requests of Muscle Withdrawal

Prior to digging into the particular energy frameworks, it's fundamental to comprehend the reason why muscles require energy and how they use it during withdrawal.

1.1 The Requirement for Energy

Cross-Scaffold Cycling: Muscle withdrawal includes the rehashed connection, turning, and separation of myosin heads to actin fibers. Each cycle requires energy as adenosine triphosphate (ATP).

Particle Siphons: Keeping up with the suitable groupings of calcium particles (Ca2+) inside and outside muscle cells requires energy-consuming particle siphons.

Unwinding: After withdrawal, muscles need energy to get back to their casual state. This cycle incorporates effectively siphoning calcium particles back into capacity.

1.2 Prompt versus Supported Energy Needs

Quick, Short-Burst Exercises: Exercises like lifting a significant burden or running require fast and significant energy creation to meet the prompt necessities of muscle compression.

Supported Exercises: Longer-span exercises like running a long distance race or cycling for expanded periods depend on more supported energy creation to give a constant stock of ATP.

Energy Frameworks in Muscle Capability

To fulfill the different energy needs of muscle capability, the body utilizes three essential energy frameworks, each with its interesting systems for ATP creation.

2.1 The Phosphagen Framework (ATP-CP Framework)

The phosphagen framework is the essential energy hotspot for short eruptions of extreme focus exercises, like lifting significant burdens or performing dangerous developments.

2.1.1 Creatine Phosphate (CP)

Creatine phosphate (CP) is a high-energy compound put away in muscle cells. It fills in as a quick wellspring of energy for the recovery of ATP during short explosions of extraordinary action.

2.1.2 Creatine Kinase

At the point when ATP is quickly drained during extreme focus work out, creatine kinase works with the exchange of a phosphate bunch from CP to adenosine diphosphate (ADP), changing over it back into ATP. This response happens rapidly and gives the energy expected to muscle compression.

2.1.3 Term of Phosphagen Framework

The phosphagen framework can support muscle withdrawal for around 10 seconds. In any case, it has restricted limit, and when CP stores are exhausted, muscles should depend on other energy frameworks to contract.

2.2 The Anaerobic Glycolytic Framework (Glycolysis)

The anaerobic glycolytic framework, otherwise called glycolysis, gives energy to exercises enduring up to around two minutes. It principally depends on glucose and glycogen put away in muscle tissue.

2.2.1 Glycolysis

Glycolysis is a progression of substance responses that separate glucose or glycogen into pyruvate, creating a modest quantity of ATP all the while. Not at all like the phosphagen framework, glycolysis doesn't need oxygen, making it a vital energy framework for exercises where oxygen conveyance is restricted.

2.2.2 Lactic Corrosive Creation

One remarkable trait of glycolysis is the development of lactic corrosive as a result. As glycolysis continues, the collection of lactic corrosive can prompt muscle weariness and inconvenience, restricting the span of anaerobic glycolytic energy creation.

2.3 The Oxygen consuming Framework (Oxidative Phosphorylation)

The oxygen consuming framework is the predominant wellspring of energy for delayed, low-to-direct power exercises enduring over two minutes. It depends on the oxidation of starches, fats, and, less significantly, proteins to deliver ATP.

2.3.1 Oxidative Phosphorylation

Oxidative phosphorylation happens inside the mitochondria of muscle cells. It includes the electron transport chain and the development of ATP from the breakdown of glucose and unsaturated fats within the sight of oxygen.

2.3.2 Fuel Sources

Carbs: Carbs as glucose and glycogen are promptly accessible and productively changed over into ATP.

Fats: Fats, put away as fatty oils, are a plentiful energy hotspot for delayed exercises and are especially significant for high-intensity games.

Proteins: In spite of the fact that proteins are not an essential energy source, they can be separated and utilized for ATP creation during delayed practice when other fuel sources are exhausted.

Transaction of Energy Frameworks

Practically speaking, these energy frameworks don't work in disengagement. They interface and cross-over, contingent upon the particular requests of the action and the accessibility of oxygen.

3.1 Introductory Energy Commitment

Phosphagen Framework: The phosphagen framework gives prompt ATP to the initial couple of moments of extreme activity.

Anaerobic Glycolytic Framework: As exercise proceeds, the anaerobic glycolytic framework turns out to be progressively significant for providing ATP.

3.2 Change to the Oxygen consuming Framework

High-impact Predominance: For longer-term exercises, the vigorous framework step by step turns into the prevailing wellspring of ATP creation, and it keeps on giving energy for however long oxygen is accessible.

Glycolytic Commitment: The glycolytic framework might in any case contribute ATP, particularly during extreme focus spans inside longer-length exercises.

3.3 Oxygen Accessibility

The accessibility of oxygen significantly impacts the decision of energy framework. Exercises acted in an oxygen-rich climate, like running or swimming, fundamentally depend on the vigorous framework. Alternately, exercises that request fast energy creation in an oxygen-drained state, such as running, vigorously draw in the anaerobic frameworks.

Elements Impacting Energy Framework Usage

A few elements impact which energy framework prevails during actual work. These variables incorporate hereditary qualities, preparing variations, sustenance, and individual wellness levels.

4.1 Hereditary Variables

People might have hereditary inclinations that make them more fit to specific kinds of proactive tasks. Hereditary varieties can impact muscle fiber piece and metabolic proficiency, at last influencing energy framework usage.

4.2 Preparation Variations

Further developed ATP-CP Framework: Obstruction preparing and extreme cardio exercise (HIIT) can improve the limit of the ATP-CP framework, taking into account more hazardous power.

Upgraded Anaerobic Glycolytic Framework: Span preparing and sport-explicit drills can work on the anaerobic glycolytic framework's capacity to create ATP without collecting unreasonable lactic corrosive.

Vigorous Perseverance: Long-term, low-to-direct power preparing, for example, distance running or cycling, can improve the high-impact framework's ability for ATP creation and oxygen usage.

4.3 Nourishment

Carbs: Sugars are the body's favored energy source, particularly during extreme focus work out. Consuming carbs previously and during activity can assist with supporting execution.

Fats: Fats give a huge wellspring of energy during lower-force, longer-length exercises. Perseverance competitors frequently depend on put away fat for fuel.

Proteins: While not an essential energy source, proteins can add to ATP creation, particularly during delayed practice when other fuel sources are exhausted.

4.4 Oxygen Accessibility

The accessibility of oxygen significantly impacts energy framework use. Exercises acted in an oxygen-rich climate, like running or swimming, fundamentally depend on the high-impact framework. Alternately, exercises that request fast energy creation in an oxygen-exhausted state, such as running, vigorously draw in the anaerobic frameworks.

Useful Applications and Execution Enhancement

Understanding energy frameworks in muscle capability has functional applications for competitors, wellness fans, and anybody looking to upgrade their actual exhibition.

5.1 Preparation Program Plan

Intense cardio exercise (HIIT): HIIT substitutes short explosions of focused energy practice with brief recuperation periods, successfully testing both the ATP-CP and anaerobic glycolytic frameworks.

Aerobic exercise: Perseverance competitors participate in longer, lower-power instructional courses to improve the oxygen consuming framework's ability.

5.2 Dietary Procedures

Sugar Stacking: Carb stacking can assist with amplifying glycogen stores before perseverance occasions.

Protein Admission: Sufficient protein consumption upholds muscle fix and can add to ATP creation during delayed work out.

Hydration: Keeping up with appropriate hydration is essential for energy framework capability and by and large execution.

5.3 Recuperation Strategies

Successful recuperation systems assist competitors with quickly returning from extreme preparation and rivalry. Strategies like extending, rub, and cryotherapy can diminish muscle irritation and backing muscle recuperation, considering better energy framework usage in ensuing meetings.

5.4 Checking and Following

Progresses in innovation have furnished competitors with apparatuses to screen and track energy framework use progressively. Wearable wellness trackers, pulse screens, and physiological testing permit people to accumulate information that can direct preparation and upgrade execution.

Clinical Ramifications and Future Headings

The comprehension of energy frameworks in muscle capability has significant clinical ramifications and opens up roads for future exploration.

6.1 Clinical Ramifications

Restoration: Information on energy frameworks is fundamental in planning recovery programs for people recuperating from wounds. Actual specialists tailor activities to modify muscle strength and capability while limiting the gamble of re-injury.

Solid Problems: Understanding energy frameworks is urgent for diagnosing and treating strong issues, for example, strong dystrophy and myasthenia gravis.

Forestalling Muscle Exhaustion: In clinical settings, overseeing muscle weariness is fundamental for patients with constant circumstances or neuromuscular problems. Strategies to limit muscle weariness can work on generally speaking personal satisfaction.

6.2 Future Bearings

Biomechanics and Mechanical technology: Investigation into muscle withdrawal mechanics illuminates the plan regarding biomechanical gadgets and automated frameworks that copy human development. These developments have applications in medical services, prosthetics, and actual restoration.

Hereditary Mediations: Advances in hereditary examination might prompt intercessions that improve energy framework productivity or alleviate muscle-related messes.

Improving Execution: As how we might interpret energy frameworks extends, we can expect more exact preparation and dietary methodologies that advance exhibition and decrease the gamble of injury.

Chapter 4

Muscle Fiber Types And Hypertrophy

Muscles are a dynamic and versatile piece of the human body, equipped for developing further and bigger through a cycle known as hypertrophy. Nonetheless, not all muscles are made equivalent, and understanding the job of muscle fiber types in hypertrophy is urgent for those trying to improve their preparation and accomplish their wellness objectives.

In this complete investigation, we will dig into the universe of muscle fiber types, looking at their qualities, capabilities, and how they connect with the hypertrophy cycle. We will likewise investigate reasonable techniques for amplifying hypertrophy in different muscle fiber types, assisting you with opening your maximum capacity in strength and size improvement.

Muscle Fiber Types

Before we plunge into the complexities of hypertrophy, understanding the various sorts of muscle strands and their special characteristics is fundamental.

1.1 Sort I (Slow-Jerk) Muscle Strands

High protection from exhaustion: Type I filaments can support withdrawals for broadened periods, making them appropriate for exercises like significant distance running or cycling.

Effective utilization of oxygen: These strands have a vigorous organization of veins (high capillarization) and a high centralization of myoglobin, a particle that works with oxygen transport inside the muscle.

Lower force creation: While Type I filaments are weariness safe, they produce less power contrasted with other fiber types.

1.2 Sort II (Quick Jerk) Muscle Filaments

1.2.1 Sort IIa Muscle Filaments

Moderate protection from weakness: Type IIa filaments have a harmony between force creation and exhaustion obstruction, making them reasonable for exercises like running and center distance running.

More noteworthy power creation: These strands produce more power than Type I filaments, making them significant for exercises requiring explosions of force.

1.2.2 Sort IIb (or IIx) Muscle Filaments

Low protection from weakness: Type IIb filaments weariness rapidly and are basically drawn in during short explosions of focused energy exercises.

High power creation: These strands are equipped for delivering critical power yet for extremely brief lengths.

1.3 Muscle Fiber Dissemination

It's vital for note that the circulation of muscle fiber types inside a singular's muscles isn't uniform. Muscles can contain differing extents of Type I, Type IIa, and Type IIb strands, which can impact a person's athletic capacities and preparing reactions.

The Study of Hypertrophy

Hypertrophy is the course of muscle development and is accomplished fundamentally by expanding the size of individual muscle strands. While hypertrophy can happen in all muscle fiber types, the degree and systems of development can contrast.

2.1 Instruments of Hypertrophy

2.1.1 Myofibrillar Hypertrophy

Myofibrillar hypertrophy includes an expansion in the size and number of myofibrils inside muscle filaments. Myofibrils contain contractile proteins (actin and myosin) liable for muscle withdrawals. Obstruction preparing, particularly with significant burdens, is a critical boost for myofibrillar hypertrophy.

2.1.2 Sarcoplasmic Hypertrophy

Sarcoplasmic hypertrophy alludes to an expansion in the volume of the sarcoplasm, the liquid filled district inside muscle filaments. The sarcoplasm contains different components, including glycogen, creatine phosphate, and mitochondria. High-reiteration opposition preparing and lifting weights style exercises are frequently connected with sarcoplasmic hypertrophy.

2.2 Fiber-Type Explicit Hypertrophy

Type II Muscle Filaments: These quick jerk strands have a higher potential for hypertrophy contrasted with Type I strands because of their more noteworthy power creating limit. Subsequently, jocks and strength competitors frequently center around hypertrophy of Type II strands.

Procedures for Muscle Fiber-Type Explicit Hypertrophy

Understanding the attributes of muscle fiber types and their reaction to preparing can assist people with fitting their gym routine schedules for explicit objectives. Here, we investigate techniques for accomplishing muscle fiber-type explicit hypertrophy.

3.1 Hypertrophy of Type I Muscle Filaments

High-Volume Preparing: Perseverance competitors frequently participate in high-reiteration, low-to-direct force opposition preparing to advance Kind I fiber hypertrophy.

Vigorous Preparation: Exercises like significant distance running, cycling, and swimming essentially draw in Type I strands, animating their development after some time.

Supported Time Under Pressure: Delayed offbeat (muscle protracting) constrictions, as found in downhill running, can prompt Sort I fiber hypertrophy.

3.2 Hypertrophy of Type II Muscle Strands

Weighty Opposition Preparing: Focused energy, low-redundancy obstruction preparing with significant burdens is a strong upgrade for Type II fiber hypertrophy. Compound activities like squats, deadlifts, and seat presses are especially compelling.

Power and Instability: Plyometric works out, Olympic lifting, and unstable developments connect with Type II strands and advance their hypertrophy.

Muscle Harm and Recuperation: Making miniature tears in muscle filaments through opposition preparing and permitting adequate recuperation time can animate Sort II fiber development.

3.3 Thorough Hypertrophy

Periodization: Organizing preparing cycles with stages committed to strength, perseverance, and power can advance complete hypertrophy.

Fluctuated Redundancy Reaches: Consolidating both high-reiteration, low-force and low-reiteration, extreme focus opposition preparing can animate development in various fiber types.

Compound and Disconnection Activities: A blend of compound developments (including various muscle gatherings) and seclusion works out (focusing on unambiguous muscles) can guarantee far reaching muscle improvement.

Nourishment and Muscle Fiber-Type Explicit Hypertrophy

Sustenance assumes a crucial part in supporting muscle hypertrophy, and different dietary techniques can supplement explicit preparation objectives in view of muscle fiber types.

4.1 Protein Admission

Type I Fiber Accentuation: Perseverance competitors might profit from a fair protein admission to help generally muscle wellbeing.

Type II Fiber Accentuation: Those focusing on Type II fiber hypertrophy ought to consider higher protein admission to work with muscle fix and development.

4.2 Starch Admission

Type I Fiber Accentuation: Perseverance competitors ought to zero in on keeping up with satisfactory carb stores (glycogen) to fuel delayed exercises.

Type II Fiber Accentuation: People focusing on Type II fiber hypertrophy might profit from sugar stacking before weighty opposition instructional courses.

4.3 Fat Admission

Type I Fiber Accentuation: Perseverance competitors might focus on an eating regimen that incorporates solid fats to help long-term work out.

Type II Fiber Accentuation: Keeping a proper equilibrium of dietary fats is essential for generally speaking wellbeing however doesn't assume an immediate part in Type II fiber hypertrophy.

Hereditary qualities, Preparing Transformations, and Muscle Fiber Types

5.1 Hereditary Elements

Hereditary elements can decide a singular's benchmark conveyance of muscle fiber types. While certain people may normally have a higher extent of Type I or Type II strands, hereditary qualities alone don't direct preparation results.

5.2 Preparation Transformations

Type I to Type II Shift: Focused energy obstruction preparing can advance a shift from Type I to Type II muscle fiber qualities, possibly expanding muscle size and strength.

Type II to Type I Shift: Aerobic exercise, like significant distance running, may prompt a shift from Type II to Type I qualities, upgrading exhaustion obstruction and perseverance.

Clinical Ramifications and Future Headings

Understanding muscle fiber types and their relationship to hypertrophy has down to earth applications in clinical settings and opens up roads for future examination.

6.1 Clinical Ramifications

Restoration: Information on muscle fiber types can illuminate restoration programs customized to a singular's particular requirements, assisting them with recuperating from wounds and recover useful limit.

Solid Problems: Understanding muscle fiber types is fundamental for diagnosing and treating muscle-related issues, for example, strong dystrophy and myasthenia gravis.

Forestalling Muscle Weariness: In clinical settings, overseeing muscle exhaustion is essential for patients with constant circumstances or neuromuscular problems. Strategies to limit muscle weakness can work on by and large personal satisfaction.

6.2 Future Headings

Hereditary Mediations: Advances in hereditary exploration might prompt mediations that improve muscle fiber type dissemination and upgrade hypertrophy potential.

Biomechanics and Advanced mechanics: Investigation into muscle constriction mechanics illuminates the plan regarding biomechanical gadgets and automated frameworks that imitate human development. These developments have applications in medical care, prosthetics, and actual recovery.

Nutrigenomics: The arising field of nutrigenomics investigates how a singular's hereditary qualities impact their reaction to eat less and work out, possibly prompting customized nourishment and preparing plans.

4.1 Understanding Muscle Fiber Types

Muscles are the motors of human development, and understanding their piece is fundamental for anyone with any interest at all in sports, wellness, or human physiology. Muscle strands, the singular cells that make up muscles, come in various kinds, each with its remarkable qualities and capabilities. In this exhaustive investigation, we will dig into the universe of muscle fiber types, analyzing their arrangements, properties, and importance with regards to athletic execution, preparing, and generally wellbeing.

Arrangement of Muscle Fiber Types

Muscle strands are extensively characterized into two primary sorts in view of their contractile properties: slow-jerk (Type I) filaments and quick jerk (Type II) strands. These arrangements are basic to understanding the variety of muscle capability in the human body.

1.1 Sluggish Jerk (Type I) Muscle Strands

Contractile Speed: These filaments contract gradually and are the most ideal for maintained, low-to-direct power exercises.

Protection from Exhaustion: Type I filaments have astounding perseverance abilities and are weariness safe, making them reasonable for long-length exercises.

Energy Creation: They basically depend on vigorous digestion, utilizing oxygen to proficiently deliver energy.

Red Tone: Type I filaments have a red appearance because of their high myoglobin content, a particle that stores and transports oxygen inside muscle cells.

Low Power Creation: While they are weakness safe, Type I filaments produce lower force contrasted with quick jerk strands.

1.2 Quick Jerk (Type II) Muscle Filaments

1.2.1 Sort IIa Muscle Strands

Moderate Speed: Type IIa strands contract at a moderate speed, offering a harmony among speed and perseverance.

Moderate Protection from Exhaustion: They have a moderate protection from weakness, making them reasonable for exercises like running and center distance running.

Energy Creation: Type IIa filaments fundamentally depend on oxygen consuming digestion yet can change to anaerobic digestion for explosions of force.

Force Creation: These strands produce more power than Type I filaments, making them significant for exercises requiring strength and power.

1.2.2 Sort IIb (or IIx) Muscle Filaments

Fast Speed: Type IIb filaments contract rapidly, making them vital for touchy developments.

Low Protection from Weakness: They exhaustion rapidly and are essentially drawn in during short eruptions of extreme focus exercises.

Energy Creation: Type IIb strands transcendently depend on anaerobic digestion to deliver energy.

Force Creation: These strands are equipped for delivering huge power yet for extremely brief lengths.

Muscle Fiber Conveyance in the Body

The conveyance of muscle fiber types inside the body isn't uniform. Various muscles contain fluctuating extents of Type I, Type IIa, and Type IIb filaments, which can impact a person's athletic capacities and preparing reactions.

2.1 Muscle-Explicit Varieties

Leg Muscles: Muscles like the quadriceps contain a higher level of Type II filaments, empowering strong developments like crouching and bouncing.

Postural Muscles: Muscles answerable for keeping up with act, like the soleus in the calf, are wealthy in Type I strands to give perseverance.

Cross breed Muscles: A few muscles, similar to the gastrocnemius in the calf, have a blend of fiber types to work with a mix of solidarity and perseverance.

2.2 Individual Fluctuation

Perseverance Competitors: People with a higher extent of Type I strands might succeed in high-intensity games like significant distance running or cycling.

Power Competitors: Those with a higher extent of Type II strands might be more qualified for power sports like running or weightlifting.

Preparing Transformations: While hereditary qualities assume a part, preparing can impact muscle fiber type circulation, permitting people to adjust to the particular requests of their picked sports or exercises.

Muscle Fiber Types and Athletic Execution

Understanding muscle fiber types is urgent for competitors and wellness devotees endeavoring to streamline their exhibition. Various games and exercises depend on unambiguous muscle fiber types to changing degrees.

3.1 High-intensity games

More prominent Weakness Opposition: Type I strands give the perseverance important to support long-length exercises.

Effective Oxygen Use: These strands have a high capillarization (vein thickness) and myoglobin content, working with productive oxygen conveyance and use.

Low Power Creation: While perseverance competitors require supported exertion, they don't depend vigorously on high power creation.

3.2 Power and Speed Sports

Fast Power Creation: Type II filaments contract rapidly and produce high power, empowering touchy developments.

Anaerobic Energy Creation: These strands essentially depend on anaerobic digestion, which gives short explosions of energy to extreme focus endeavors.

Exhaustion Obstruction: Type IIa strands, with a harmony between speed and perseverance, are urgent for exercises like center distance running and running.

3.3 Half breed Sports and Exercises

Group activities: Sports like soccer, ball, and football include a blend of running, perseverance, and power developments, requiring a decent circulation of muscle fiber types.

Useful Preparation: Utilitarian wellness preparing integrates various developments, making it vital to foster a balanced muscle structure with a blend of fiber types.

Preparing Techniques for Muscle Fiber Types

Preparing systems can be custom fitted to target explicit muscle fiber types, assisting people with enhancing their presentation in different games and exercises.

4.1 Sort I Fiber Accentuation

High-Volume Preparing: Participate in high-redundancy, low-to-direct power obstruction preparing to advance Kind I fiber hypertrophy.

High-impact Preparing: Take part in lengthy term, low-power exercises like significant distance running or cycling to draw in and animate Sort I strands.

Supported Time Under Pressure: Delayed unusual (muscle extending) withdrawals, like downhill running, can prompt Sort I fiber hypertrophy.

4.2 Sort II Fiber Accentuation

Weighty Obstruction Preparing: Consolidate extreme focus, low-reiteration opposition preparing with significant burdens to animate Kind II fiber hypertrophy. Compound activities like squats, deadlifts, and seat presses are especially successful.

Power and Dangerousness: Incorporate plyometric works out, Olympic lifting, and unstable developments to connect with Type II strands and advance their hypertrophy.

Muscle Harm and Recuperation: Make miniature tears in muscle filaments through obstruction preparing and permit adequate recuperation time to animate Kind II fiber development.

4.3 Thorough Muscle Advancement

Periodization: Construction preparing cycles with stages committed to strength, perseverance, and ability to advance exhaustive muscle improvement.

Changed Reiteration Reaches: Consolidate both high-redundancy, low-power and low-reiteration, extreme focus opposition preparing to animate development in various fiber types.

Compound and Separation Activities: Join compound developments (including numerous muscle gatherings) and segregation works out (focusing on unambiguous muscles) to guarantee balanced muscle advancement.

Sustenance and Muscle Fiber Types

5.1 Protein Admission

Protein is fundamental for muscle development and fix. Competitors can change their protein consumption in view of their preparation center:

Type I Fiber Accentuation: Perseverance competitors might profit from a decent protein admission to help generally speaking muscle wellbeing.

Type II Fiber Accentuation: Those focusing on Type II fiber hypertrophy ought to consider higher protein admission to work with muscle fix and development.

5.2 Starch Admission

Type I Fiber Accentuation: Perseverance competitors ought to zero in on keeping up with sufficient carb stores (glycogen) to fuel delayed exercises.

Type II Fiber Accentuation: People focusing on Type II fiber hypertrophy might profit from carb stacking before weighty obstruction instructional meetings.

5.3 Fat Admission

Type I Fiber Accentuation: Perseverance competitors might focus on an eating regimen that incorporates sound fats to help long-length work out.

Type II Fiber Accentuation: Keeping a proper equilibrium of dietary fats is essential for in general wellbeing yet doesn't assume an immediate part in Type II fiber hypertrophy.

Muscle Fiber Types and Maturing

The arrangement of muscle fiber types can change with age, and understanding these movements is significant for keeping up with muscle wellbeing and capability in later years.

6.1 Age-Related Changes

Type II Fiber Decline: More seasoned grown-ups frequently experience a decrease in Type II muscle filaments, prompting diminished power and strength.

Type I Fiber Conservation: Type I filaments will quite often be more safeguarded with maturing, adding to perseverance and postural steadiness.

Practical Ramifications: Changes in muscle fiber types can affect a singular's capacity to perform day to day exercises and keep up with generally personal satisfaction.

6.2 Opposition Preparing and Maturing

Hypertrophy: Opposition preparing advances muscle hypertrophy, especially in Type II strands, assisting more established grown-ups with keeping up with strength and practical limit.

Balance: Further developing muscle strength and equilibrium through obstruction preparing can lessen the gamble of falls and wounds in more established people.

Generally Wellbeing: Customary obstruction preparing can add to by and large wellbeing and prosperity in maturing populaces.

4.2 Muscle Hypertrophy and Growth Mechanisms

Muscles are an exceptional and versatile piece of the human body, equipped for developing further and bigger through an interaction known as hypertrophy. Whether you're a competitor intending to upgrade your presentation, a weight lifter taking a stab at noteworthy muscle gains, or somebody trying to work on their general wellbeing and body, understanding the instruments behind muscle hypertrophy is fundamental. In this complete investigation, we will dive into the study of muscle development, analyzing the cell cycles, factors, and reasonable techniques that drive hypertrophy.

The Study of Muscle Hypertrophy

Prior to jumping into the complexities of muscle hypertrophy, understanding the major science behind it is fundamental.

1.1 What Is Muscle Hypertrophy?

Muscle hypertrophy is the most common way of expanding the size and mass of individual muscle filaments, eventually prompting a broadening of the whole muscle. It happens because of explicit physiological upgrades, essentially opposition preparing or strength-based works out.

1.2 Components of Muscle Hypertrophy

1.2.1 Myofibrillar Hypertrophy

Myofibrillar hypertrophy is portrayed by an expansion in the size and number of myofibrils inside muscle filaments. Myofibrils are the contractile parts of muscle cells containing actin and myosin fibers, which empower muscle compressions. Obstruction preparing with significant burdens is a critical upgrade for myofibrillar hypertrophy.

1.2.2 Sarcoplasmic Hypertrophy

Sarcoplasmic hypertrophy alludes to an expansion in the volume of the sarcoplasm, the liquid filled locale inside muscle strands. The sarcoplasm contains different components, including glycogen, creatine phosphate, and mitochondria. High-redundancy opposition preparing and lifting weights style exercises are frequently connected with sarcoplasmic hypertrophy.

Cell Systems of Muscle Hypertrophy

To acquire a more profound knowledge into muscle hypertrophy, investigating the cell processes that drive this wonderful transformation is fundamental.

2.1 Muscle Fiber Enrollment

Type I (Slow-Jerk) Muscle Strands: These are enrolled first and basically utilized during low-force, perseverance type exercises.

Type II (Quick Jerk) Muscle Strands: These filaments are selected as the force of the activity increments. Type II filaments are additionally separated into Type IIa and Type IIb (or IIx) strands, with Type IIb being enrolled last and fundamentally drew in during focused energy endeavors.

2.2 Mechanical Strain

Mechanical strain, the power produced during muscle compressions against obstruction, is a basic calculate muscle hypertrophy. Heavier loads and obstruction make more noteworthy mechanical strain, prompting myofibrillar hypertrophy.

2.3 Muscle Harm

Opposition preparing can cause miniature tears in muscle strands, starting a maintenance and development process. This muscle harm triggers aggravation and the arrival of development factors, for example, insulin-like development factor (IGF-1), which add to muscle hypertrophy.

2.4 Metabolic Pressure

Metabolic pressure happens during high-reiteration, lower-weight obstruction preparing. It prompts the gathering of metabolic side-effects like lactate and hydrogen particles, which are accepted to assume a part in invigorating hypertrophy, particularly sarcoplasmic hypertrophy.

Elements Affecting Muscle Hypertrophy

Various variables add to the degree and pace of muscle hypertrophy. Understanding these variables permits people to improve their preparation and nourishment methodologies.

3.1 Preparation Factors

Power: Focused energy opposition preparing with significant burdens is especially compelling for myofibrillar hypertrophy.

Volume: High preparation volume, accomplished through different sets and redundancies, can add to both myofibrillar and sarcoplasmic hypertrophy.

Recurrence: Steady and standard instructional courses are fundamental for muscle development.

Practice Determination: Compound activities that draw in numerous muscle gatherings, like squats and deadlifts, are successful for generally speaking muscle improvement.

3.2 Sustenance

Caloric Excess: To help muscle development, people frequently need to consume a larger number of calories than they use (caloric excess).

Protein Admission: Protein is fundamental for muscle fix and development. Satisfactory protein admission is critical for hypertrophy.

Starches: Carbs give energy to exercises and assist with recharging muscle glycogen stores, supporting preparation force.

Fats: Sound fats assume a part in chemical creation and generally wellbeing yet don't straightforwardly add to muscle hypertrophy.

3.3 Chemicals

Testosterone: Testosterone is a strong anabolic chemical that advances muscle development. Opposition preparing can increment testosterone levels for a brief time.

Development Chemical (GH): GH invigorates the arrival of IGF-1 and assumes a part in muscle fix and development.

Insulin-Like Development Element 1 (IGF-1): IGF-1 is delivered because of GH and adds to muscle development and fix.

Cortisol: Cortisol, a pressure chemical, can catabolically affect muscle tissue. Overseeing pressure and upgrading recuperation is critical to control cortisol levels.

Reasonable Methodologies for Muscle Hypertrophy

To accomplish huge muscle hypertrophy, people can execute pragmatic methodologies that consolidate preparing, sustenance, and recuperation.

4.1 Moderate Over-burden

Expanding loads lifted

Adding more sets and reiterations

Decreasing rest periods between sets

Fluctuating activity power and intricacy

4.2 Changed Redundancy Reaches

Low redundancies (1-5) with significant burdens for myofibrillar hypertrophy

Moderate redundancies (6-12) for an equilibrium of hypertrophy types

High reiterations (12+) with lighter loads for sarcoplasmic hypertrophy

4.3 Periodization

Hypertrophy Stage: Focuses on muscle development with higher-volume, moderate-weight lifting.

Strength Stage: Spotlights on expanding maximal strength with lower-redundancy, higher-power lifting.

Deloading Stage: Gives recuperation and forestalls overtraining.

4.4 Recuperation and Rest

Rest: Guarantee quality rest for ideal recuperation and chemical guideline.

Nourishment: Consume a decent eating routine wealthy in protein, starches, and fats to help muscle fix.

Dynamic Recuperation: Consolidate low-force exercises like strolling or yoga on rest days to help recuperation.

Muscle Hypertrophy and Age

Muscle hypertrophy isn't restricted to youthful competitors; it stays applicable as people age. Truth be told, it turns out to be progressively significant for keeping up with generally speaking wellbeing and utilitarian limit.

5.1 Sarcopenia

Sarcopenia is the age-related loss of bulk and strength, which can prompt diminished versatility and expanded hazard of falls and cracks. Obstruction preparing and muscle hypertrophy systems can help neutralize sarcopenia.

5.2 Hormonal Changes

As people age, hormonal changes, for example, diminished testosterone and development chemical levels, can influence muscle support and development. Obstruction preparing and legitimate nourishment become basic for safeguarding bulk and capability.

5.3 Utilitarian Advantages

Portability and autonomy

Bone wellbeing

Metabolic wellbeing

Equilibrium and fall counteraction

Chapter 5

Strength Training Principles

Strength preparing is a basic part of actual wellness that has various advantages, from expanding bulk and capacity to working on bone thickness and by and large wellbeing. To leave on a powerful strength preparing venture, understanding the central rules that guide the process is urgent. In this thorough investigation, we will dig into the science and craft of solidarity preparing, looking at the key rules that support its prosperity, the physiological components included, and commonsense procedures for accomplishing your solidarity objectives.

Understanding Strength Preparing

Prior to digging into the standards of solidarity preparing, we should lay out a reasonable comprehension of what strength preparing is and its significance.

1.1 What Is Strength Preparing?

Free loads: Hand weights, hand weights, and portable weights.

Opposition machines: Leg squeezes, chest presses, and link machines.

Bodyweight works out: Push-ups, pull-ups, and squats.

1.2 Significance of Solidarity Preparing

Muscle Development: Advances muscle hypertrophy, expanding muscle size and definition.

Expanded Strength: Upgrades actual strength, making regular assignments more straightforward.

Worked on Bone Wellbeing: Animates bone thickness, diminishing the gamble of osteoporosis.

Metabolic Advantages: Lifts digestion, supporting weight the executives.

Injury Avoidance: Fortifies connective tissues and balances out joints, lessening the gamble of wounds.

Utilitarian Limit: Improves practical limit with regards to day to day exercises and athletic execution.

Standards of Solidarity Preparing

Presently, how about we investigate the crucial rules that oversee powerful strength preparing programs.

2.1 Moderate Over-burden

The rule of moderate over-burden is the underpinning of solidarity preparing. It includes steadily expanding the obstruction or responsibility after some time to challenge the muscles ceaselessly. This dynamic test invigorates muscle development and strength gains.

Step by step instructions to Apply Moderate Over-burden:

Increment the weight lifted as you become more grounded.

Add more sets and redundancies to your exercises.

Decline rest periods between sets to increase exercises.

Fluctuate practice force and intricacy.

2.2 Explicitness

The guideline of explicitness expresses that preparing transformations are intended for the sort of preparing performed. With regards to strength preparing, this implies that the activities, developments, and obstruction utilized ought to intently match your solidarity objectives.

Instructions to Apply Explicitness:

Pick practices that focus on the muscle bunches you need to reinforce.

Adjust your preparation to your particular exhibition objectives (e.g., powerlifting, working out, useful strength).

2.3 Overtraining and Recuperation

Offsetting preparing force with sufficient recuperation is pivotal. Overtraining, or not permitting adequate recuperation, can prompt burnout, wounds, and slowed down progress. Recuperation incorporates rest days, legitimate sustenance, and satisfactory rest.

Instructions to Execute Recuperation:

Plan rest days between serious exercises.

Focus on rest and hold back nothing long periods of value rest.

Consume a reasonable eating regimen wealthy in protein, sugars, and sound fats to help muscle fix and development.

2.4 Variety and Periodization

To forestall levels and upgrade progress, integrating variety into your preparation is fundamental. Periodization includes sorting out preparing into explicit stages, each with its concentration, power, and objectives.

Step by step instructions to Apply Variety and Periodization:

Change activities, sets, and redundancies consistently.

Cycle between strength, hypertrophy, and perseverance stages.

Plan deloading weeks to take into account recuperation and forestall overtraining.

2.5 Appropriate Method and Structure

Executing practices with appropriate strategy and structure is crucial for wellbeing and viability. Unfortunate structure can prompt wounds and breaking point progress.

The most effective method to Keep up with Appropriate Procedure and Structure:

Look for direction from a certified mentor or mentor.

Begin with lighter loads to learn appropriate structure.

Center around controlled and purposeful developments.

Use mirrors or video criticism to survey structure.

2.6 Individualization

Strength preparing projects ought to be custom-made to individual objectives, capacities, and impediments. What works for one individual may not work for another.

Instructions to Individualize Preparing:

Survey your assets, shortcomings, and objectives.

Think about any wounds or actual constraints.

Adjust activities and preparing factors to suit your necessities.

Physiological Instruments of Solidarity Preparing

Understanding the physiological instruments behind strength preparing can develop your appreciation for the interaction and guide your preparation systems.

3.1 Muscle Hypertrophy

Myofibrillar Hypertrophy: Includes an expansion in the size and number of myofibrils inside muscle filaments, prompting expanded contractile power.

Sarcoplasmic Hypertrophy: Includes an expansion in the volume of the sarcoplasm, the liquid filled area inside muscle filaments, prompting more prominent energy stockpiling and perseverance.

3.2 Brain Variations

Strength acquires in the underlying phases of preparing frequently result from brain variations, as opposed to huge muscle development. These transformations incorporate better engine unit enlistment, expanded engine neuron terminating rates, and improved engine coordination.

3.3 Hormonal Reactions

Testosterone: A vital chemical for muscle development and strength, testosterone levels normally increment after opposition preparing.

Development Chemical (GH): GH animates the arrival of insulin-like development factor (IGF-1), adding to muscle fix and development.

Cortisol: While cortisol is catabolic (separating tissue), transient increments during preparing are ordinary and help with energy assembly.

3.4 Muscle Fiber Enlistment

Type I (Slow-Jerk) Filaments: Connected with during low-power, perseverance type exercises.

Type II (Quick Jerk) Filaments: Connected as exercise power increments. Type II filaments are additionally separated into Type IIa and Type IIb (or IIx) strands, with Type IIb being selected last and essentially drew in during focused energy endeavors.

Pragmatic Systems for Successful Strength Preparing

Developing an effective fortitude preparation program requires a smart methodology that integrates these standards into your daily schedule.

4.1 Objective Setting

Begin by characterizing clear, sensible objectives. Is it true that you are holding back nothing, bulk, or both? Could it be said that you are preparing for a particular game or movement? Laying out unambiguous objectives will assist you with fitting your program.

4.2 Activity Determination

4.3 Preparation Recurrence

Decide how frequently you'll prepare each muscle bunch. Fledglings can begin with 2-3 meetings each week, while cutting edge lifters might profit from 4-6 meetings.

4.4 Redundancies and Sets

Strength: Lower redundancies (1-5) with significant burdens.

Hypertrophy: Moderate redundancies (6-12) with moderate loads.

Perseverance: Higher redundancies (12+) with lighter loads.

4.5 Movement

Reliably increment the opposition or power of your exercises to apply the rule of moderate over-burden. Keep a preparation log to keep tabs on your development.

4.6 Recuperation

Focus on recuperation through rest, sustenance, and rest. Overtraining can thwart progress, so pay attention to your body and take into account adequate recuperation between exercises.

Normal Legends and Confusions

As you set out on your solidarity preparing venture, it's fundamental to know about normal fantasies and misinterpretations that can thwart your advancement.

5.1 Fantasy: Ladies Will Get Massive from Strength Preparing

This legend isn't accurate. Strength preparing can assist ladies with developing slender muscle and increment fortitude without causing unreasonable cumbersomeness. The degree of muscle development generally relies upon hereditary qualities, nourishment, and preparing power.

5.2 Legend: Strength Preparing Is Just for the Youthful

Strength preparing is helpful for people, all things considered. More seasoned grown-ups, specifically, can utilize strength preparing to keep up with bulk, work on bone thickness, and improve practical limit.

5.3 Fantasy: You Really want an Exercise center Participation to Strength Train

While admittance to a rec center gives an assortment of gear, viable strength preparing should likewise be possible at home or outside utilizing bodyweight works out, opposition groups, or straightforward family things.

5.4 Legend: Strength Preparing Is Hazardous

When performed with legitimate strategy and under management, strength preparing is a protected and compelling type of activity. Look for direction from a certified mentor or mentor in the event that you're uncertain about your structure.

5.1 Progressive Overload

Moderate over-burden is the key rule that supports fruitful strength preparing and muscle advancement. It is the foundation of any compelling preparation program, whether you're a fledgling hoping to develop a strong underpinning of fortitude or an accomplished competitor taking a stab at constant improvement. In this exhaustive investigation, we will dive into the idea of moderate over-burden, figure out its importance, investigate the science behind it, and give commonsense methodologies to integrate it into your preparation schedule.

Figuring out Moderate Over-burden

1.1 Characterizing Moderate Over-burden

Moderate over-burden is a preparation idea that includes deliberately and slowly expanding the pressure or obstruction put on the body during exercise. The objective is to challenge the muscles and other physiological frameworks past their ongoing limit, driving them to adjust and become more grounded after some time.

1.2 The Meaning of Moderate Over-burden

Animating Muscle Development: It is the essential component for muscle hypertrophy, the most common way of expanding muscle size.

Strength Improvement: Moderate over-burden prompts more noteworthy strength gains by reliably stretching the boundaries of your muscles.

Forestalling Levels: Without moderate over-burden, preparing levels can happen, and progress might slow down.

Productivity: It guarantees that your exercises stay successful and effective, prompting ceaseless enhancements.

Injury Counteraction: By progressively expanding obstruction, it lessens the gamble of abuse wounds related with unexpected, unreasonable burden increments.

1.3 The Science Behind Moderate Over-burden

To comprehend the reason why moderate over-burden works, it's fundamental to inspect the physiological components included.

1.3.1 Muscle Fiber Enlistment

At the point when you take part in opposition preparing, your body initiates muscle filaments in a particular request. At first, it actuates more modest, lower-limit engine units, essentially made out of sluggish jerk (Type I) muscle strands. As the opposition or power increments, bigger, higher-edge engine units with quick jerk (Type II) muscle strands are enrolled.

Slow-Jerk Muscle Filaments: Utilized for lower-power, perseverance exercises.

Quick Jerk Muscle Strands: Connected with for extreme focus, power-arranged endeavors.

Moderate over-burden guarantees that you consistently challenge your muscles by requiring the enrollment of more muscle strands, incorporating those with more prominent development potential (quick jerk filaments).

1.3.2 Muscle Hypertrophy

Myofibrillar Hypertrophy: Includes the development and variation of myofibrils, the contractile units inside muscle strands. This prompts expanded strength and power.

Sarcoplasmic Hypertrophy: Includes the extension of the sarcoplasm, the liquid filled area inside muscle filaments. It upgrades energy capacity and perseverance.

Moderate over-burden sets off these transformations as the interest for force age and energy creation inside muscle cells increments.

Carrying out Moderate Over-burden

Now that we comprehend the importance and study of moderate over-burden, we should investigate reasonable techniques for its successful execution.

2.1 Put forth Clear Objectives

Prior to setting out on a strength preparing program, lay out clear and explicit objectives. Whether your goal is to increment bulk, further develop strength, upgrade perseverance, or accomplish a mix of these, having clear cut objectives will direct your preparation plan.

2.2 Select Suitable Activities

Pick practices that line up with your objectives and draw in the objective muscle bunches really. Compound activities, like squats, deadlifts, seat presses, and lines, are fantastic decisions for by and large strength advancement.

2.3 Control Obstruction

Expanding Weight: Progressively increment the weight lifted as your solidarity moves along. This can include adding more weight plates to a free weight, utilizing heavier free weights, or changing the opposition on practice machines.

Adding Redundancies: Increment the quantity of reiterations you perform for a given activity. For instance, in the event that you were completing three arrangements of 10 reiterations, progress to three arrangements of 12 redundancies.

Counting Extra Sets: Integrate more arrangements of an activity to increment preparing volume. Rather than three sets, you could do four or five arrangements of a specific activity.

Diminishing Rest Periods: Abbreviate the rest time frames between sets to make your exercises really testing. This can strengthen the preparation upgrade and advance transformation.

Shifting Activities: Change between various varieties of an activity to give new difficulties to your muscles. For example, you can switch back and forth between free weight squats and free weight jumps for lower-body preparing.

2.4 Periodization

Periodization is the efficient preparation of a preparation program to improve execution and forestall levels. It includes isolating your preparation into unmistakable stages, each with explicit objectives and force levels.

Hypertrophy Stage: Spotlights on expanding muscle size and normally includes moderate loads and higher redundancies.

Strength Stage: Focuses on working on maximal strength with lower reiterations and heavier loads.

Power Stage: Accentuates the advancement of hazardous strength and speed.

Deloading Stage: Gives recuperation and lessens preparing force to forestall overtraining and advance recuperation.

Periodization guarantees that you cycle through various preparation stages, forestalling variation levels and consistently testing your muscles.

2.5 Screen Progress

Keeping tabs on your development is fundamental for carrying out moderate over-burden really. Keep a preparation diary to record your exercises, including the activities, loads utilized, reiterations, and sets performed. This record permits you to see your enhancements over the long haul and make informed acclimations to your preparation plan.

2.6 Pay attention to Your Body

While moderate over-burden is fundamental, it's similarly critical to pay attention to your body and focus on security. Keep away from overtraining, which can prompt wounds and burnout. Assuming you experience determined agony or distress, it's urgent to rest, recuperate, and look for proficient direction if important.

Moderate Over-burden in Various Preparation Modalities

Moderate over-burden can be applied to different preparation modalities, including weightlifting, bodyweight preparing, and cardiovascular activity.

3.1 Weightlifting

In weightlifting, moderate over-burden principally includes expanding the obstruction or weight utilized for works out. This can be accomplished by steadily adding weight to free weights or free weights or changing opposition on weight machines.

3.2 Bodyweight Preparing

For bodyweight works out, moderate over-burden can be accomplished by controlling factors like reiterations, sets, and exercise varieties. As you become more capable, you can build the test by performing more troublesome varieties of bodyweight practices or adding weight vests or obstruction groups.

3.3 Cardiovascular Activity

Indeed, even in cardiovascular activity, moderate over-burden can be applied. You can expand the power of your cardio exercises by:

Speeding up: Run, cycle, or swim at a quicker pace.

Hoisting Grade: Use slant settings on treadmills or slope surfaces for uphill running or strolling.

Expanding Span: Step by step broaden the length of your cardio meetings to build the preparation boost.

Moderate Over-burden and Nourishment

While moderate over-burden is basically connected with work out, nourishment assumes a significant part in supporting muscle development and in general execution.

4.1 Caloric Excess

To work with muscle development, consuming an adequate number of calories is fundamental. A slight caloric excess, where you consume a bigger number of calories than you exhaust, gives the energy expected to muscle fix and development.

4.2 Protein Admission

Protein is the structure block of muscle tissue. Sufficient protein admission is fundamental for muscle fix and development. Expect to consume an adequate measure of excellent protein sources in your eating regimen.

4.3 Carbs and Fats

Carbs give the energy expected to extraordinary instructional meetings, while fats assume a part in chemical creation and generally speaking wellbeing. Guarantee a decent admission of both macronutrients to help your preparation endeavors.

4.4 Hydration

Appropriate hydration is basic for ideal execution. Drying out can adversely affect strength and perseverance, so guarantee you stay satisfactorily hydrated previously, during, and after your exercises.

5.2 Periodization

Periodization is an efficient and vital way to deal with preparing that has upset the manner in which competitors and wellness devotees plan and design their exercises. It includes separating the preparation cycle into particular stages, each with explicit objectives and power levels. Periodization is a flexible instrument that can be applied to different games, wellness objectives, and expertise levels, assisting people with accomplishing maximized operation, forestall burnout, and ceaselessly progress. In this

exhaustive investigation, we will dig into the idea of periodization, its standards, types, and functional systems to execute it really in your preparation routine.

Figuring out Periodization

1.1 Characterizing Periodization

Periodization is a preparation procedure that partitions the general preparation plan into more modest, coordinated, and sensible stages or periods. Every period has a particular concentration, force level, and span, with a definitive objective of upgrading athletic execution or accomplishing explicit wellness targets.

1.2 The Advancement of Periodization

The idea of periodization has a rich history, with establishes in Eastern European games science and training rehearses. Dr. Leonid Matveyev, a Russian games researcher, is frequently credited with creating periodization standards during the twentieth 100 years. After some time, periodization has advanced and acquired notoriety across different games and wellness spaces.

1.3 The Significance of Periodization

Forestalling Overtraining: By cycling between various preparation stages, it takes into consideration sufficient recuperation and forestalls overtraining, lessening the gamble of wounds and burnout.

Upgrading Execution: It guarantees that competitors top with impeccable timing, performing at their best during contests.

Persistent Movement: Periodization advances steady improvement by testing the body with changing upgrades.

Improving Inspiration: Breaking the preparation year into sensible periods can keep competitors spurred, as they pursue explicit, reachable objectives.

Variation and Recuperation: It recognizes the body's requirement for transformation and recuperation, which is fundamental for long haul achievement.

Standards of Periodization

Successful periodization is directed by a bunch of basic rules that direct the way in which preparing cycles are organized and executed.

2.1 Moderate Over-burden

The guideline of moderate over-burden, examined exhaustively in a past article, is at the center of periodization. Each preparing stage ought to step by step increment in force to challenge the body and animate transformation. This is accomplished by controlling factors like obstruction, volume, and power.

2.2 Particularity

The guideline of particularity underscores fitting preparation to match the particular requests of the game or wellness objective. In periodization, this implies that each stage ought to focus on the physiological and expertise prerequisites of the impending occasion or objective.

2.3 Variety

Variety guarantees that preparing stays intriguing and successful. It includes intermittently evolving works out, preparing modalities, and power levels inside each stage to forestall variation levels and keep up with progress.

2.4 Individualization

Preparing plans ought to be individualized in light of the competitor's one of a kind qualities, including wellness level, objectives, qualities, shortcomings, and recuperation limit. Customization guarantees that the periodization plan is viable and feasible.

2.5 Periodization Periods

Macrocycle: The longest preparation cycle, frequently spreading over a year or a serious season. It is partitioned into mesocycles.

Mesocycle: Moderate stages, generally enduring half a month to a while, zeroing in on unambiguous preparation goals (e.g., hypertrophy, strength, power).

Microcycle: The briefest preparation cycle, commonly enduring multi week, that frames consistent exercise schedules and activities.

Kinds of Periodization

There are a few periodization models, each with its remarkable design and accentuation. We should investigate probably the most broadly utilized types.

3.1 Direct Periodization

Direct periodization is a customary model that advances through particular stages in a straight style. It normally begins with a high-volume, low-force stage and slowly changes

to bring down volume and higher power as the preparation cycle advances. This approach considers consistent movement and is many times utilized in sports with obvious serious seasons, such as powerlifting.

3.2 Non-Direct Periodization

Non-direct periodization, otherwise called undulating periodization, presents more successive changes in power and volume inside more limited time spans. Rather than following a straight movement, it includes vacillations in preparing factors all through the preparation week or month. Non-straight periodization is reasonable for competitors who lean toward assortment in their exercises and can be especially viable for muscle hypertrophy and in general wellness.

3.3 Block Periodization

Block periodization isolates the preparation year into particular blocks, each zeroing in on a particular preparation viewpoint, like hypertrophy, strength, or power. Each block might most recent half a month, and the accentuation on one preparation viewpoint permits competitors to expand transformations. Block periodization is exceptionally versatile and can be redone for various games and objectives.

3.4 Form Periodization

Form periodization, promoted by Louie Simmons and utilized in powerlifting and strength sports, consolidates different preparation strategies in a solitary preparation cycle. It integrates various kinds of lifts, including max exertion and dynamic exertion lifts, to upgrade strength, power, and speed. This approach underlines persistent assortment and difficulties the body with various upgrades.

3.5 Triphasic Periodization

Triphasic periodization, created by Cal Dietz, separates preparing into three essential stages: offbeat, isometric, and concentric. Each stage focuses on a particular part of solidarity and power improvement. Triphasic periodization is especially advantageous for competitors trying to work on their hazardousness and athletic execution.

Functional Utilization of Periodization

Now that we've investigated the standards and sorts of periodization, how about we examine how to apply it to your preparation routine basically.

4.1 Put forth Clear Objectives

Begin by characterizing your preparation goals. Whether you want to increment strength, construct muscle, further develop perseverance, or upgrade sports execution, having clear and explicit objectives will direct your periodization plan.

4.2 Make a Preparation Schedule

Plan your preparation year or cutthroat season by outlining macrocycles and mesocycles. Recognize contest dates or maximized execution periods and work in reverse to decide when explicit stages ought to start and end.

4.3 Stage Construction

Inside each mesocycle, structure your preparation stages as indicated by your objectives. For instance, a strength-centered stage might incorporate activities like squats and deadlifts, while a power-centered stage might consolidate unstable developments like cleans or plyometrics.

4.4 Movement

Carry out the rule of moderate over-burden by progressively expanding force, volume, or intricacy inside each stage. This might include adding weight to works out, expanding the quantity of reiterations or sets, or shortening rest spans.

4.5 Checking and Changes

Consistently survey your advancement by following execution measurements, for example, strength gains, body structure changes, or sports-explicit upgrades. Change your preparation plan depending on the situation in view of your perceptions and criticism from mentors or coaches.

4.6 Recuperation and Deloading

Integrate booked rest and deloading periods into your preparation intend to guarantee legitimate recuperation and forestall overtraining. These periods permit your body to adjust and supercompensate, prompting further developed execution in resulting stages.

4.7 Sustenance and Periodization

Sustenance assumes an essential part in supporting periodized preparing. Tailor your eating regimen to match the particular requests of each preparing stage. For example, during a hypertrophy stage, center around adequate protein consumption and caloric excess to help muscle development.

6

Chapter 6

Nutrition and Muscular Strength

Sustenance assumes a vital part in our general wellbeing and prosperity, however its importance is enhanced with regards to solid strength. Solid strength isn't just fundamental for actual execution yet in addition for keeping up with useful autonomy and forestalling wounds. This article investigates the multifaceted connection among nourishment and strong strength, diving into the key supplements, dietary systems, and way of life factors that can improve muscle advancement and execution. Whether you're a competitor taking a stab at max execution or a singular hoping to keep up with bulk and strength, understanding the science behind sustenance and strong strength is significant.

1. **The Essentials of Solid Strength**
   1.1 Meaning of Strong Strength
   Strong strength alludes to the greatest power a muscle or gathering of muscles can produce in a solitary withdrawal. It is a fundamental part of actual wellness and is expected for different day to day exercises, sports, and work-out schedules. Strong strength is generally estimated utilizing tests like the one-reiteration greatest (1RM), which decides the most extreme weight an individual can

lift for one redundancy of a given activity.

1.2 Significance of Solid Strength

Strong strength isn't just about having protruding biceps yet additionally about utilitarian strength that upholds exercises of day to day living. It helps with keeping up with great stance, forestalling wounds, and working on by and large actual execution. In addition, it turns out to be progressively critical as we age, as it can assist with neutralizing muscle misfortune (sarcopenia) and keep up with autonomy.

2. The Job of Nourishment in Strong Strength

2.1 Protein: The Structure Block of Muscles

Protein is many times called the structure block of muscles, and justifiably. It comprises of amino acids, the fundamental parts for muscle fix, development, and upkeep. To expand solid strength, it's fundamental to consume a satisfactory measure of top notch protein sources, like lean meats, fish, dairy items, eggs, and plant-based choices like tofu and vegetables. The suggested everyday protein consumption for people hoping to construct muscle is around 1.2 to 2.2 grams of protein per kilogram of body weight.

2.2 Starches: Powering Muscle Execution

Sugars are the body's essential energy source, particularly during extreme focus exercises. Consuming a satisfactory measure of carbs guarantees that your muscles have sufficient glycogen stores to help your exercises. Low-carb diets can prompt muscle exhaustion and frustrate strength gains. Complex carbs like entire grains, organic products, and vegetables ought to be focused on in your eating regimen.

2.3 Fats: Fundamental for Chemical Creation

While sugars give speedy energy, fats assume a critical part in chemical creation, including chemicals like testosterone, which are imperative for muscle development. Sound fats from sources like avocados, nuts, seeds, and greasy fish ought to be remembered for a fair eating routine.

2.4 Micronutrients: Supporting Muscle Capability

Vitamin D: It supports calcium ingestion, which is significant for muscle constrictions. Normal wellsprings of vitamin D incorporate daylight, greasy fish, and strengthened food sources.

Calcium: Other than being significant for bone wellbeing, calcium is associated with muscle compression. Dairy items, salad greens, and invigorated food sources are brilliant sources.

Magnesium: This mineral is vital for muscle unwinding after withdrawals. It very well may be tracked down in nuts, seeds, entire grains, and salad greens.

Iron: Iron inadequacy can prompt weariness, influencing your capacity to actually prepare. Great wellsprings of iron incorporate red meat, poultry, beans, and strengthened grains.

3. Dietary Techniques for Amplifying Strong Strength

3.1 Feast Timing

Timing your feasts around your exercises can essentially influence your solid strength gains. Consuming a fair feast with a blend of protein and carbs 2-3 hours before exercise can give the fundamental energy and supplements. Moreover, a post-exercise feast or tidbit, preferably in something like two hours after work out, assists with muscle recuperation and development.

3.2 Protein Appropriation

As opposed to stacking up on protein in one dinner, conveying your protein consumption over the course of the day is useful. This approach guarantees a consistent inventory of amino acids for muscle fix and development. Plan to remember a wellspring of protein for every dinner and tidbit.

3.3 Hydration

Legitimate hydration is frequently neglected yet is fundamental for solid strength. Parchedness can prompt muscle squeezes and diminished execution. Hydrate reliably over the course of the day, and consider sports drinks with electrolytes during extraordinary exercises to supplant lost liquids and minerals.

3.4 Supplement Timing

Supplement timing alludes to the essential utilization of supplements (particularly protein and starches) around your exercises. A few competitors and jocks practice supplement timing, consuming a protein and carb rich feast or shake preceding or after an exercise to upgrade muscle development and recuperation.

4. Macronutrient Proportions and Strong Strength

4.1 High-Protein Diets

High-protein abstains from food have acquired notoriety among those hoping to amplify solid strength and hypertrophy (muscle development). These eating regimens ordinarily comprise of 20-35% of day to day calorie consumption from protein sources. While high-protein diets can be successful for muscle constructing, offsetting them with sufficient starches and fats for generally wellbeing and performance is fundamental.

4.2 Sugar Stacking

Sugar stacking is a procedure regularly utilized by perseverance competitors, yet it can likewise help people engaged with extreme focus, strength-centered exercises. By expanding sugar consumption in the days paving the way to a major instructional course or contest, you can guarantee your glycogen stores are completely loaded for ideal execution.

4.3 Sound Fats

Remembering sound fats for your eating routine is essential for chemical equilibrium and generally wellbeing. While fats ought not be the essential wellspring of calories for muscle building, they assume a strong part in keeping up with energy levels and advancing recuperation.

5. Supplements and Solid Strength

5.1 Protein Enhancements

Protein supplements, like whey protein, casein protein, and plant-based choices like pea protein, can be advantageous wellsprings of protein for people battling to meet their day to day needs through entire food sources alone. These enhancements are frequently utilized as post-exercise shakes to help muscle recuperation.

5.2 Creatine

Creatine is one of the most widely read up and successful enhancements for working on strong strength and power. It recovers adenosine triphosphate (ATP), the essential energy cash of cells, taking into account more extreme and supported muscle constrictions. Creatine monohydrate is the most explored structure and is ok for most people.

5.3 Expanded Chain Amino Acids (BCAAs)

BCAAs, including leucine, isoleucine, and valine, are fundamental amino acids that assume a part in muscle protein blend and diminishing muscle irritation. They are normally tracked down in protein-rich food sources but at the same time are accessible in supplement structure for those looking for designated help.

5.4 Beta-Alanine

Beta-alanine is an amino corrosive that can improve strong perseverance by buffering the development of lactic corrosive during extraordinary activity. It's not unexpected found in pre-exercise supplements and may assist people with pushing through focused energy instructional meetings.

5.5 Nutrient and Mineral Enhancements

While it's ideal to get fundamental nutrients and minerals from entire food sources, a few people might profit from supplementation, especially assuming they have explicit lacks that influence solid strength. Counseling a medical care proficient for customized guidance is fundamental.

6. Way of life Variables and Strong Strength

6.1 Rest

Sufficient rest is essential for muscle recuperation and development. During profound rest organizes, the body discharges development chemical, which assumes a huge part in fixing and building muscle tissue. Go for the gold long stretches of value rest each evening.

6.2 Pressure The board

Ongoing pressure can prompt muscle catabolism (breakdown) and upset strength gains. Integrate pressure decrease strategies like contemplation, profound breathing, or yoga into your daily schedule to help muscle wellbeing.

6.3 Obstruction Preparing

Obstruction preparing, like weightlifting or bodyweight works out, is the essential upgrade for muscle development and strength advancement. A very much planned opposition preparing program that dynamically expands the power of activities is fundamental for long haul strength gains.

6.4 Rest and Recuperation

Muscles need time to fix and develop after extreme exercises. Overtraining can prompt muscle weakness and even injury. Integrate rest days into your preparation plan and focus on recuperation methodologies, for example, froth rolling, extending, and rub.

7. **The Effect Old enough on Strong Strength and Sustenance**
7.1 Age-Related Muscle Misfortune

As people age, they normally experience a decrease in bulk and strength, a peculiarity known as sarcopenia. Legitimate nourishment turns out to be considerably more basic in more established grown-ups to neutralize this misfortune. Satisfactory protein consumption, joined with opposition preparing, can assist with relieving age-related muscle decline.

7.2 Unique Contemplations for More seasoned Grown-ups

More established grown-ups may have different nourishing requirements and difficulties, for example, decreased hunger, trouble biting, or gulping. In such cases, working with an enrolled dietitian can assist with fostering a tweaked nourishment plan that resolves these issues and supports strong strength.

8. Normal Fantasies and Misinterpretations

8.1 Protein Overconsumption

A typical misinterpretation is that consuming unnecessary protein prompts bigger muscles. Truly, the body can involve a specific measure of protein for muscle building, and overabundance protein is processed or put away as fat. A fair protein admission is a higher priority than over the top utilization.

8.2 Spot Decrease

Another legend is that designated activities can diminish fat in unambiguous region of the body. While obstruction preparing can fabricate muscle in unambiguous regions, fat misfortune happens all through the body with a blend of a reasonable eating regimen and generally calorie consumption.

9. Contextual investigations and Examples of overcoming adversity

9.1 Competitor Examples of overcoming adversity

Looking at the dietary and preparing regimens of fruitful competitors can give significant experiences into the job of nourishment in accomplishing solid strength. Contextual analyses of competitors who have created critical additions through sustenance and preparing changes can rouse and illuminate perusers.

6.1 Role of Macronutrients (Proteins, Carbs, Fats)

Nourishment is the underpinning of good wellbeing, and macronutrients are the fundamental parts of our eating routine that give us energy and imperative supplements. These macronutrients incorporate proteins, starches, and fats, each with remarkable jobs and works in keeping up with our prosperity. In this exhaustive investigation, we will dig into the meaning of each macronutrient, their sources, and how they add to our general wellbeing.

1. Proteins: The Structure Blocks of Life

1.1 Definition and Construction

Proteins are complicated particles comprised of amino acids, which are frequently alluded to as the "building blocks of life." There are 20 unique amino acids, and their plan in a protein's design decides its capability. Proteins are fundamental for the development, fix, and support of tissues, catalysts, chemicals, and the safe framework.

1.2 Wellsprings of Protein

Protein-rich food varieties come from both creature and plant sources. Creature sources incorporate meat, poultry, fish, eggs, and dairy items. Plant-based protein sources incorporate vegetables (beans, lentils, chickpeas), tofu, tempeh, nuts, seeds, and grains (quinoa, bulgur, and farro).

1.3 Job in Wellbeing

Muscle Building and Fix: Amino acids from dietary proteins are fundamental for muscle development and fix, making them fundamental for competitors and people participating in normal activity.

Compound Capability: Numerous catalysts that work with synthetic responses in the body are proteins.

Safe Framework Backing: Antibodies, which shield against diseases, are proteins.

Chemical Guideline: Chemicals like insulin and development chemical are protein-based and direct different physical processes.

Underlying scaffolding: Collagen, a primary protein, gives solidarity to our skin, bones, and connective tissues.

2. **Sugars: The Body's Essential Energy Source**
   2.1 Definition and Types

Sugars are the body's essential wellspring of energy. They are partitioned into three primary sorts: sugars, starches, and dietary fiber. Sugars are basic carbs found in food sources like natural products, honey, and table sugar. Starches are perplexing sugars found in food varieties like grains, vegetables, and vegetables. Dietary fiber, likewise a mind boggling starch, is tracked down in organic products, vegetables, entire grains, and vegetables and is fundamental for stomach related wellbeing.

2.2 Wellsprings of Carbs

Grains: Rice, wheat, oats, grain, and corn.

Vegetables: Beans, lentils, peas, and chickpeas.

Organic products: Apples, bananas, oranges, and berries.

Vegetables: Broccoli, carrots, spinach, and yams.

Sugars: Sucrose (table sugar), fructose (tracked down in organic products), and lactose (tracked down in dairy items).

2.3 Job in Wellbeing

Energy Creation: Carbs are changed over into glucose, which gives energy to cells and powers our everyday exercises.

Mind Capability: Glucose is the essential fuel for the cerebrum, supporting mental capabilities and mental clearness.

Stomach related Wellbeing: Dietary fiber helps processing, controls glucose levels, and advances a sensation of completion.

Muscle Glycogen: Starches are put away in the muscles as glycogen, which is utilized during active work.

Glucose Guideline: Fiber-rich starches assist with balancing out glucose levels, lessening the gamble of diabetes.

3. Fats: Fundamental for Wellbeing

3.1 Definition and Types

Fats, otherwise called lipids, are fundamental macronutrients that give a concentrated wellspring of energy. There are different kinds of fats, including soaked fats, unsaturated fats, and trans fats. Unsaturated fats can be additionally isolated into monounsaturated and polyunsaturated fats. While soaked fats are normally strong at room temperature (e.g., spread), unsaturated fats are fluid (e.g., olive oil).

3.2 Wellsprings of Fats

Creature Fats: Meat, poultry, greasy fish (salmon, mackerel), dairy items, and eggs.

Plant Fats: Avocado, nuts (almonds, pecans), seeds (flaxseeds, chia seeds), olive oil, and coconut oil.

3.3 Job in Wellbeing

Energy Capacity: Fat is an exceptionally productive energy stockpiling particle, permitting the body to store overabundance energy for sometime in the future.

Cell Design: Fats are essential parts of cell layers, guaranteeing appropriate cell capability.

Protection: Subcutaneous fat gives protection and controls internal heat level.

Ingestion of Fat-Solvent Nutrients: Fat is important for the retention of fat-solvent nutrients (A, D, E, and K).

Chemical Creation: Cholesterol, a kind of fat, is a forerunner to steroid chemicals like testosterone and estrogen.

4. Adjusting Macronutrients for Ideal Wellbeing

4.1 The Significance of a Decent Eating routine

Ideal wellbeing depends on the right equilibrium of macronutrients. A decent eating routine guarantees that the body gets the vital supplements for energy, development, and upkeep while lessening the gamble of ongoing sicknesses.

4.2 Macronutrient Proportions

The ideal macronutrient proportion changes relying upon individual objectives, movement levels, and medical issue. Normal macronutrient proportions include:

Adjusted Diet: Around 45-65% of absolute everyday calories from sugars, 10-35% from protein, and 20-35% from fats.

High-Protein Diet: A higher protein consumption, for example, 30-40% of day to day calories, is frequently prescribed for competitors and those hoping to construct muscle.

Low-Carb Diet: A lower carb consumption, around 20-50 grams each day, is normal in low-carb eats less like keto.

Low-Fat Eating regimen: Low-fat weight control plans intend to keep fat admission under 20-30% of everyday calories, frequently suggested for heart wellbeing.

4.3 Individualized Nourishment

Nourishing necessities fluctuate extraordinarily among people, so it's vital to consider individual factors, for example, age, orientation, movement level, and explicit ailments while deciding macronutrient proportions. Counseling an enrolled dietitian or medical services proficient can give customized direction.

5. The Effect of Macronutrients on Weight The board

5.1 Weight reduction and Weight Gain

The equilibrium of macronutrients in your eating regimen can essentially affect your weight the executives objectives. For weight reduction, a calorie deficiency (consuming less calories than you consume) is fundamental. This can be accomplished by lessening in general calorie admission, which frequently includes directing sugar and fat admission while guaranteeing a satisfactory protein admission to protect bulk.

5.2 Satiety and Craving Control

Protein and dietary fiber are known for their satisfying properties, helping you feel full and fulfilled. Counting these macronutrients in your feasts can uphold craving control and lessen generally speaking calorie utilization.

5.3 Close to home and Careful Eating

Understanding the close to home and mental parts of eating is likewise essential for weight the executives. Perceiving profound triggers for gorging and rehearsing careful eating can supplement macronutrient balance in accomplishing and keeping a sound weight.

6. Macronutrients and Ongoing Sickness

6.1 Heart Wellbeing

Dietary fats, especially soaked and trans fats, can affect heart wellbeing. High admission of immersed and trans fats is related with an expanded gamble of coronary illness. Supplanting soaked and trans fats with unsaturated fats, like those tracked down in olive oil, nuts, and greasy fish, can decidedly affect cardiovascular wellbeing.

6.2 Diabetes The executives

Carbs straightforwardly influence glucose levels, making carb the board fundamental for people with diabetes. Complex carbs with a low glycemic file (GI) are liked as they slowerly affect glucose. Also, solid fats and fiber can assist with balancing out glucose levels.

6.3 Weight-Related Conditions

Corpulence and metabolic disorder are connected to imbalanced macronutrient utilization. An eating routine that advances a decent admission of starches, protein, and fats, joined with segment control, normal activity, and way of life changes, can help oversee and forestall these circumstances.

6.2 Micronutrients and Hydration

Micronutrients and hydration are two fundamental parts of a solid eating routine that frequently get less consideration than macronutrients (proteins, starches, and fats). Nonetheless, these micronutrients, including nutrients and minerals, as well as legitimate hydration, assume a basic part in keeping up with ideal wellbeing and prosperity. In this extensive investigation, we will dig into the meaning of micronutrients and hydration, their sources, capabilities, and their effect on our general wellbeing.

1. **Micronutrients: The Supplement Forces to be reckoned with**
   1.1 Definition and Types
   Micronutrients are fundamental nutrients and minerals expected by the body in little amounts for different physiological capabilities. They can be sorted into two fundamental gatherings: fat-dissolvable and water-solvent.

   Fat-Solvent Nutrients: These nutrients, including A, D, E, and K, are dissolvable in fat and can be put away in the body for broadened periods. They are fundamental for different capabilities, like vision, bone wellbeing, and blood thickening.

Water-Solvent Nutrients: This gathering incorporates L-ascorbic acid and the B-complex nutrients (B1, B2, B3, B5, B6, B7, B9, B12). These nutrients break down in water and are not put away in huge sums, making ordinary dietary admission fundamental.

1.2 Wellsprings of Micronutrients

Vitamin A: Found in food sources like yams, carrots, spinach, and liver.

Vitamin D: Daylight openness and dietary sources like greasy fish, braced dairy items, and eggs.

Vitamin E: Nuts, seeds, vegetable oils, and salad greens.

Vitamin K: Salad greens, broccoli, and liver.

L-ascorbic acid: Citrus organic products, berries, peppers, and kiwi.

B-Complex Nutrients: Tracked down in different food varieties, including entire grains, meat, dairy items, and mixed greens.

1.3 Job in Wellbeing

Invulnerable Capability: Nutrients and minerals like L-ascorbic acid, vitamin D, and zinc support the resistant framework, assisting the body with warding off contaminations.

Bone Wellbeing: Calcium and vitamin D are urgent for solid bones and forestalling conditions like osteoporosis.

Energy Creation: B-complex nutrients are fundamental for energy digestion, helping convert food into usable energy.

Vision: Vitamin An is imperative for keeping up with great vision and forestalling night visual impairment.

Cell reinforcement Safeguard: Nutrients C and E, as well as minerals prefer selenium and zinc, go about as cell reinforcements, shielding cells from harm brought about by free revolutionaries.

2. **The Significance of Legitimate Hydration**

2.1 Definition and Importance

Hydration alludes to the most common way of keeping an ideal equilibrium of water in the body. Satisfactory hydration is crucial for generally speaking wellbeing and is associated with different physical processes, including temperature guideline, assimilation, dissemination, and the disposal of side-effects.

2.2 Wellsprings of Hydration

Water: Plain water is awesome and most direct wellspring of hydration.

Drinks: Other hydrating refreshments incorporate home grown teas, clear stocks, and weakened organic product juices.

Leafy foods: Many products of the soil have high water content, like watermelon, cucumber, and lettuce.

2.3 Job in Wellbeing

Temperature Guideline: Sweat is the body's cooling instrument, and satisfactory hydration guarantees proficient temperature guideline, particularly during actual work or warm climate.

Processing: Water helps in the breakdown of food and the retention of supplements in the stomach related framework.

Flow: Blood is for the most part made out of water, and sufficient hydration guarantees the effective vehicle of oxygen and supplements to cells.

Detoxification: Water upholds the disposal of side-effects and poisons from the body through pee and sweat.

Mental Capability: Lack of hydration can debilitate mental capability, influencing concentration, focus, and memory.

3. Micronutrient and Hydration Associations

3.1 Micronutrients and Hydration

Sodium: Sodium is an electrolyte that directs liquid equilibrium in the body. Consuming a suitable measure of sodium is fundamental for keeping up with hydration.

Potassium: Potassium works couple with sodium to adjust liquid levels in cells. It likewise assumes a part in muscle constrictions and nerve capability.

Magnesium: Magnesium upholds muscle and nerve capability, including the guideline of muscle constrictions, which is pivotal for keeping up with legitimate hydration.

3.2 Micronutrient Lacks and Hydration

Calcium: Deficient calcium admission might prompt muscle spasms and influence the body's capacity to keep up with legitimate liquid equilibrium.

Vitamin D: Vitamin D is engaged with calcium assimilation, by implication affecting hydration.

Potassium and Magnesium: Lacks in these minerals can prompt muscle shortcoming and spasms, possibly influencing hydration status.

4. Keeping up with Micronutrient and Hydration Equilibrium

4.1 Dietary Wellsprings of Micronutrients and Hydration

A fair eating routine wealthy in different food varieties is the best method for guaranteeing satisfactory admission of the two micronutrients and hydration. An eating routine that incorporates organic products, vegetables, entire grains, lean proteins, and dairy items can give fundamental nutrients, minerals, and water.

4.2 Micronutrient Enhancements

While an even eating routine ought to give most micronutrients, a few people might expect enhancements to address explicit lacks. Nonetheless, it's fundamental to talk with a medical services supplier or enrolled dietitian prior to taking enhancements, as unreasonable admission can be unsafe.

4.3 Hydration Needs

Hydration needs fluctuate from one individual to another and are affected by variables, for example, age, action level, environment, and by and large wellbeing. An overall principle is to go for the gold 10 cups (64-80 ounces) of water each day, however individual necessities might vary. Thirst is a solid sign of hydration needs, and it's fundamental to pay attention to your body.

4.4 Parchedness Anticipation

Hydrate routinely over the course of the day, particularly in hot or sticky circumstances.

Focus on thirst signs and drink when you feel parched.

Limit caffeine and liquor utilization, as they can prompt expanded liquid misfortune.

Eat water-rich food sources like products of the soil.

Screen pee tone; light yellow demonstrates appropriate hydration, while dim yellow might flag drying out.

5. Micronutrient Lacks and Wellbeing Suggestions

5.1 Nutrient and Mineral Insufficiencies

Lack of vitamin D: Can prompt bone problems, debilitated safe capability, and expanded powerlessness to contaminations.

Lack of iron: Results in frailty, portrayed by weariness, shortcoming, and diminished oxygen-conveying limit of the blood.

L-ascorbic acid Insufficiency (Scurvy): Causes exhaustion, muscle shortcoming, joint agony, and gum dying.

Lack of vitamin A: Can prompt night visual deficiency and an expanded gamble of contaminations.

Iodine Lack: May bring about thyroid problems and formative issues.

5.2 Wellbeing Outcomes of Drying out

Gentle Parchedness: Side effects incorporate dry mouth, expanded thirst, dull pee, and weariness.

Moderate Lack of hydration: May cause tipsiness, fast heartbeat, dry skin, and diminished pee yield.

Serious Lack of hydration: Can bring about disarray, indented eyes, quick breathing, and swooning, requiring prompt clinical consideration.

6.3 Supplements for Strength

Supplements have become progressively famous among competitors, jocks, and wellness devotees hoping to upgrade their solidarity, muscle development, and by and

large execution. While legitimate nourishment and preparing are the establishment for developing fortitude, enhancements can supplement these endeavors by giving explicit supplements and mixtures that help muscle advancement, recuperation, and execution. In this exhaustive investigation, we will dive into the universe of enhancements for strength, examining their adequacy, security, and the job they play in accomplishing ideal outcomes.

1. **Protein Enhancements**
   1.1 Whey Protein
   Whey protein is one of the most famous enhancements for strength and muscle development. It is a finished protein, wealthy in fundamental amino acids, especially leucine, which assumes a pivotal part in muscle protein combination. Whey protein is quickly consumed by the body, settling on it an optimal decision for post-exercise recuperation. It gives the fundamental amino acids to muscle fix and development, particularly when consumed inside the "anabolic window" after work out.

   1.2 Casein Protein
   Casein protein is another dairy-based protein supplement that is more slow to process contrasted with whey. This sluggish processing can be invaluable, particularly before sleep time, as it gives a consistent arrival of amino acids over the course of the evening, advancing muscle recuperation during rest. A few people likewise utilize a mix of whey and casein for a fair protein consumption.

   1.3 Plant-Based Protein
   For the people who follow a veggie lover or vegetarian diet, plant-based protein supplements offer an option in contrast to creature determined proteins. Sources like pea protein, earthy colored rice protein, and hemp protein can give sufficient protein admission important to muscle development. These enhancements are frequently joined to make a total amino corrosive profile.

2. **Creatine**
   2.1 Creatine Monohydrate
   Creatine is one of the most widely explored and demonstrated supplements for improving strength and power. It works by

expanding the body's store of phosphocreatine, which recovers adenosine triphosphate (ATP), the essential energy cash of cells. This considers more quick and supported muscle withdrawals during extreme focus exercises, like weightlifting and running. Various examinations have shown the way that creatine supplementation can prompt huge strength gains, especially in practices that include short explosions of energy, for example, seat presses, squats, and deadlifts. Creatine monohydrate is the most explored and generally suggested type of creatine.

2.2 Measurements and Timing

An ordinary creatine stacking stage includes requiring 20 grams each day (split into four dosages) for 5-7 days, trailed by a support period of 3-5 grams each day. Timing can change, yet numerous competitors like to take creatine following their exercise, close by a starch source, to upgrade retention.

2.3 Security

Creatine is by and large thought to be protected when taken inside suggested portions. Nonetheless, people with kidney infection or other prior ailments ought to counsel a medical care proficient prior to utilizing creatine. Remaining enough hydrated while taking creatine is additionally fundamental to forestall potential secondary effects like muscle cramps.

3. Stretched Chain Amino Acids (BCAAs)

3.1 Definition and Sythesis

Stretched chain amino acids (BCAAs) allude to three fundamental amino acids: leucine, isoleucine, and valine. These amino acids are extraordinary in light of the fact that they are used principally in muscle tissue as opposed to the liver, making them an expected wellspring of energy during exercise. BCAAs are remembered to advance muscle protein amalgamation, decrease muscle irritation, and forestall muscle breakdown during serious exercises.

3.2 Advantages for Strength and Recuperation

Muscle Recuperation: BCAAs might decrease muscle irritation and speed up the recuperation interaction, taking into consideration more regular, extreme instructional courses.

Muscle Protein Blend: Leucine, specifically, assumes a fundamental part in starting muscle protein combination, making it a fundamental part of BCAA supplements.

Energy Protection: During delayed exercises, BCAAs can be utilized as an energy source, possibly postponing muscle exhaustion.

3.3 Dose and Timing

The suggested measurement of BCAAs changes, however a typical reach is 5-20 grams each day, regularly taken previously, during, or after exercises. Timing can differ contingent upon individual inclinations and preparing objectives.

4. Beta-Alanine

4.1 Definition and System of Activity

Beta-alanine is a normally happening amino corrosive that consolidates with histidine in the body to shape carnosine. Carnosine goes about as a cradle, assisting with diminishing the development of lactic corrosive in muscles during extraordinary activity. This buffering impact postpones the beginning of muscle exhaustion and permits competitors to push through extreme focus instructional meetings.

4.2 Advantages for Strength and Perseverance

Expanded Muscle Perseverance: Beta-alanine can work on the capacity to perform more reiterations in obstruction preparing, which might prompt more noteworthy strength gains.

Upgraded Anaerobic Execution: It can improve execution in exercises requiring short eruptions of focused energy exertion, for example, running and weightlifting.

Postponed Exhaustion: By lessening the gathering of lactic corrosive, beta-alanine might defer the beginning of muscle weariness during extraordinary exercises.

4.3 Dose and Timing

The common dose for beta-alanine is 3-6 grams each day,

separated into more modest portions to limit the "shivering" sensation (paresthesia) that a few people insight. Taking beta-alanine close by a feast can likewise assist with lessening this incidental effect.

5. **Nitric Oxide Supporters**

5.1 Definition and Component of Activity

Nitric oxide (NO) is a particle that loosens up veins, taking into consideration expanded blood stream. Supplements known as nitric oxide supporters, frequently containing fixings like L-arginine and L-citrulline, are accepted to upgrade blood stream to muscles during exercise. This expanded blood stream might convey more oxygen and supplements to muscle tissue, possibly further developing strength and perseverance.

5.2 Advantages for Strength and Execution

Nitric oxide sponsors are regularly used to improve athletic execution and may offer the accompanying advantages:

Expanded Muscle Siphon: Numerous competitors report an impermanent expansion in muscle "siphon" or completion during exercises, which can add to inspiration and saw strength gains.

Further developed Perseverance: Upgraded blood stream might assist muscles with getting through longer during obstruction and cardiovascular preparation.

Potential for Expanded Strength: While research on strength gains from NO supporters is restricted, a few people report further developed strength execution.

5.3 Measurement and Timing

Measurements of nitric oxide sponsors can differ contingent upon the particular fixings and item. Normal doses for L-arginine territory from 2 to 6 grams each day, while L-citrulline is frequently taken at dosages of 3 to 6 grams each day. Timing ordinarily includes taking the enhancement 30-an hour prior to work out.

6. **Security Contemplations and Expected Aftereffects**

6.1 General Security

Counsel a Medical services Proficient: Prior to starting any new enhancement routine, particularly in the event that you have basic medical issue or are taking meds, counsel a medical services proficient.

Quality Matters: Pick respectable brands and items that have gone through testing for virtue and quality.

Screen for Aftereffects: Know about any antagonistic impacts related with enhancements and end use if vital.

6.2 Possible Secondary effects

Creatine: A few people might encounter gastrointestinal uneasiness or muscle cramps.

Beta-Alanine: Paresthesia (shivering sensation) is a typical incidental effect, particularly with high portions.

Nitric Oxide Promoters: Potential aftereffects might incorporate stomach related issues and cerebral pains.

6.3 Individual Variety

It's fundamental to perceive that singular reactions to enhancements can fluctuate. What functions admirably for one individual might not affect another. Beginning with lower portions and progressively expanding can assist with surveying individual resistance and limit possible incidental effects.

Chapter 7

Recovery and Performance Optimization

Recuperation and execution advancement are two unpredictably connected parts of making athletic progress and keeping up with by and large prosperity. In this thorough investigation, we will dive profound into the universe of recuperation methodologies and execution upgrade procedures, revealing insight into their importance, viability, and their essential job in assisting people with accomplishing their maximum capacity in sports, wellness, and day to day existence.

1. The Significance of Recuperation
1.1 Characterizing Recuperation
Recuperation is the cycle by which the body fixes, remakes, and adjusts following activity or stress. It incorporates a scope of physical and mental techniques that assist the body with getting back to a condition of equilibrium and status for future endeavors. Appropriate recuperation is fundamental for execution advancement, injury counteraction, and long haul prosperity.
1.2 The Recuperation Cycle
Quick Post-Exercise: Chilling off, extending, and renewing liquids.

Transient Recuperation: Supplement admission, rest, and limiting irritation.

Long haul Recuperation: Sufficient rest, dynamic recuperation, and stress the executives.

2. **The Job of Sustenance in Recuperation**

2.1 Macronutrients and Micronutrients

Sustenance assumes a focal part in the recuperation cycle. Satisfactory admission of macronutrients (proteins, starches, and fats) and micronutrients (nutrients and minerals) is essential for muscle fix, energy renewal, and generally recuperation.

Proteins: Fundamental for muscle fix and development, proteins give the important amino acids expected to remake tissues harmed during exercise.

Starches: Carbs renew glycogen stores, giving energy to ensuing exercises and helping with recuperation.

Fats: Sound fats support chemical creation and decrease irritation, adding to the recuperation cycle.

Nutrients and Minerals: Micronutrients assume different parts in recuperation, including cell reinforcement guard and resistant help.

2.2 Hydration

Appropriate hydration is fundamental for recuperation, as it helps transport supplements to cells, manages internal heat level, and flushes out side-effects. Lack of hydration can block recuperation and prevent execution.

2.3 Timing and Supplement Proportions

Timing and supplement proportions are basic variables in recuperation nourishment. Consuming a decent dinner with a mix of macronutrients inside the post-work out "anabolic window" (30 minutes to 2 hours) can upgrade recuperation. Protein-to-sugar proportions, for example, 3:1 or 4:1, are generally prescribed to help muscle fix and glycogen recharging.

3. Rest and Recuperation

3.1 The Job of Rest

Quality rest is a foundation of recuperation and execution improvement. During profound rest organizes, the body discharges development chemical, which is fundamental for muscle fix and development. Rest likewise upholds mental capability, mind-set guideline, and resistant framework capability.

3.2 Rest Cleanliness

Keep a Reliable Rest Timetable: Heading to sleep and awakening simultaneously every day manages your body's interior clock.

Make a Loosening up Sleep time Schedule: Participating in quieting exercises before rest, like perusing or contemplation, can advance better rest quality.

Enhance Rest Climate: Guarantee your room is dull, calm, and at an agreeable temperature to establish an optimal dozing climate.

4. Dynamic Recuperation Techniques

4.1 Definition and Advantages

Lessening Muscle Irritation: Delicate developments can assist with mitigating muscle solidness and touchiness.

Upgrading Blood Stream: Expanded course conveys supplements to muscles and eliminate byproducts.

Mental Unwinding: Dynamic recuperation exercises like yoga or comfortable strolling can advance unwinding and stress decrease.

4.2 Instances of Dynamic Recuperation Exercises

Yoga: Yoga advances adaptability, unwinding, and stress decrease while connecting with muscles in a delicate way.

Swimming: Swimming is a low-influence movement that gives cardiovascular advantages and advances muscle recuperation.

Strolling or Light Running: A relaxed walk or light run can invigorate blood stream and decrease muscle snugness.

5. Inactive Recuperation Procedures

5.1 Definition and Advantages

Muscle Fix: Rest considers more effective muscle fix and development.

Chemical Equilibrium: Sufficient rest upholds hormonal equilibrium, including development chemical and testosterone.

Mental Recuperation: Aloof recuperation gives mental and profound recovery, decreasing pressure and advancing in general prosperity.

5.2 Instances of Uninvolved Recuperation Procedures

Rest and Rest: Focus on helpful rest and take into consideration additional rest days when required.

Back rub and Bodywork: Proficient back rubs or self-myofascial discharge strategies can decrease muscle pressure and advance unwinding.

Reflection and Care: Practices like contemplation and profound breathing can assist with diminishing pressure and work on mental recuperation.

6. Supplements for Recuperation

6.1 Protein Enhancements

Protein supplements, like whey protein, casein protein, and plant-based protein, can be gainful for post-practice recuperation. They give fundamental amino acids important to muscle fix and development, particularly when entire food protein sources are not promptly accessible.

6.2 Stretched Chain Amino Acids (BCAAs)

BCAAs, including leucine, isoleucine, and valine, can assist with diminishing muscle irritation and advance muscle protein combination. BCAA supplements are much of the time consumed during or after exercises to help recuperation and diminish work out incited muscle harm.

6.3 Omega-3 Unsaturated fats

Omega-3 unsaturated fats, found in fish oil supplements, have calming properties that can help with decreasing activity actuated irritation and muscle touchiness. Omega-3 supplementation may likewise uphold joint wellbeing and generally recuperation.

6.4 Collagen Enhancements

Collagen is a protein that offers underlying help to connective tissues, including ligaments, tendons, and skin. Collagen enhancements might assist with supporting joint wellbeing and diminish the gamble of injury by fortifying connective tissues.

6.5 Cell reinforcements

Cancer prevention agent supplements, like nutrients C and E, as well as minerals can imagine zinc and selenium, can assist with killing free revolutionaries delivered during exercise. This can decrease oxidative pressure and aggravation, supporting recuperation and lessening muscle harm.

7. Mental Recuperation

7.1 Pressure The board

Stress the board is a vital part of recuperation and execution streamlining. Elevated degrees of stress, whether from preparing, work, or day to day existence, can adversely affect physical and mental prosperity. Procedures for stress the executives incorporate contemplation, care, profound breathing activities, and unwinding methods.

7.2 Representation and Mental Symbolism

Representation and mental symbolism strategies include intellectually practicing and imagining effective exhibitions. Competitors frequently utilize these strategies to upgrade concentration, certainty, and mental availability.

7.3 Objective Setting and Arranging

Putting forth clear and reachable objectives, both present moment and long haul, can give inspiration and course. Arranging and organizing preparing and recuperation plans assist competitors with remaining coordinated and improve their presentation.

8. Execution Enhancement Techniques

8.1 Periodization

Periodization is an orderly way to deal with preparing that includes separating the preparation year into particular stages, each with explicit objectives and forces. This approach forestalls overtraining, advance recuperation, and upgrade execution over the long run.

8.2 Broadly educating

Broadly educating includes participating in various types of activity or sports to adjust actual requests and decrease the gamble of abuse wounds. It can likewise give mental reward and advance by and large wellness.

8.3 Biomechanical Examination

Biomechanical examination includes evaluating a competitor's development examples and method to distinguish regions for development. This examination can assist with advancing execution and diminish the gamble of injury by refining structure and proficiency.

9. Execution Following and Checking

9.1 Preparation Logs

Keeping a preparation log permits competitors to keep tabs on their development, including exercises, recuperation systems, and execution measurements. A preparation log can assist with distinguishing examples and changes required for ceaseless improvement.

9.2 Wearable Innovation

Headways in wearable innovation, for example, wellness trackers and pulse screens, empower competitors to screen different physiological boundaries, including pulse, rest

quality, and recuperation status. These devices give important information to upgrading preparing and recuperation systems.

9.3 Blood Tests

A few competitors go through standard blood testing to evaluate supplement levels, hormonal equilibrium, and generally wellbeing. Blood tests can assist with distinguishing lacks or lopsided characteristics that might influence recuperation and execution.

7.1 Importance of Rest and Recovery

In our speedy and requesting world, rest and recuperation are much of the time underestimated parts of a solid way of life. In any case, they are essential parts of keeping up with physical, mental, and close to home prosperity. Whether you are a competitor looking for max execution or a singular taking a stab at generally speaking wellbeing, understanding the significance of rest and recuperation is fundamental. In this exhaustive investigation, we will dig into the meaning of rest and recuperation, how they add to our wellbeing, and down to earth methodologies for integrating them into our lives.

1. **Actual Recuperation**

   1.1 Muscle Recuperation

   Rest is fundamental for the body's normal cycles of muscle fix and development. After active work or exercise, muscle tissues experience miniature tears and weakness. Satisfactory rest permits these tissues to mend, recover, and become more grounded. Non-stop strain without adequate rest can prompt abuse wounds and upset progress in strength preparing or athletic execution.

   1.2 Glycogen Rebuilding

   During exercise, the body drains its glycogen stores, which are the essential wellspring of energy for extreme focus exercises. Rest, alongside legitimate sustenance, empowers glycogen to be recharged in muscles and the liver. This guarantees that you have the energy saves fundamental for future exercises and supported active work.

   1.3 Chemical Guideline

   Rest, a critical part of rest, assumes a urgent part in hormonal equilibrium. Chemicals like development chemical, testosterone, and cortisol are delivered and managed during various phases of rest. Development chemical, specifically, helps with muscle recuperation and tissue fix. Predictable, quality rest guarantees legitimate hormonal capability, supporting actual recuperation.

2. Mental Recuperation

2.1 Mental Capability

Rest isn't only fundamental for the body; it is similarly essential for the brain. Consistent mental requests, for example, business related pressure or extraordinary mental concentration, can prompt mental weariness and diminished mental execution. Brief breaks and satisfactory rest permit the mind to recuperate and keep up with ideal mental capability.

2.2 Memory Combination

Rest, especially REM (quick eye development) rest, assumes a central part in memory solidification. During this stage, the cerebrum cycles and stores data from the day. Deficient rest can debilitate memory maintenance, fixation, and critical thinking skills.

2.3 Pressure Decrease

Rest and unwinding strategies, for example, contemplation and care, assist with lessening pressure and advance mental recuperation. Persistent pressure can prompt profound fatigue, nervousness, and burnout. Integrating supportive practices into day to day existence can moderate the adverse impacts of pressure and work on mental prosperity.

3. Close to home Recuperation

3.1 Profound Flexibility

Rest adds to close to home versatility by permitting people to process and recuperate from inner difficulties. Helpful exercises, such as investing energy with friends and family, seeking after side interests, or basically having some time off, support close to home recuperation and develop profound fortitude.

3.2 Mind-set Guideline

Satisfactory rest and unwinding assume a urgent part in temperament guideline. Lack of sleep and persistent pressure can prompt mind-set aggravations, including crabbiness, temperament swings, and sadness. Focusing on rest keeps up with close to home equilibrium and psychological wellness.

4. The Resistant Framework

4.1 Resistant Capability

Rest and rest are firmly connected to resistant capability. During profound rest, the body creates and delivers cytokines, a kind of protein that assumes a part in safe reaction and irritation control. Quality rest upholds a powerful insusceptible framework, diminishing the gamble of contaminations and diseases.

4.2 Fiery Reaction

Constant lack of sleep and deficient rest can prompt an overactive fiery reaction in the body. This ongoing aggravation is related with different ailments, including cardiovascular sickness, diabetes, and immune system problems. Rest and rest assist with directing the body's incendiary cycles, advancing long haul wellbeing.

5. Systems for Integrating Rest and Recuperation

5.1 Rest Cleanliness

Keep a reliable rest plan by heading to sleep and awakening simultaneously consistently, even on ends of the week.

Establish an agreeable rest climate with a strong sleeping pad, proper room temperature, and insignificant light and commotion.

Try not to invigorate exercises before sleep time, for example, screen time or extraordinary activity.

Limit caffeine and liquor consumption, particularly in the hours paving the way to rest.

Practice unwinding methods like profound breathing or contemplation to quiet the brain before rest.

5.2 Helpful Exercises

Integrating helpful exercises into day to day existence can advance physical, mental, and close to home recuperation:

Plan standard breaks during work or study meetings to rest and re-energize.

Take part in side interests and exercises that give pleasure and unwinding, like perusing, planting, or craftsmanship.

Invest quality energy with friends and family and construct social associations, which can offer close to home help and improve prosperity.

Investigate unwinding procedures like moderate muscle unwinding, yoga, or care reflection.

5.3 Dynamic Recuperation

Consolidate low-power exercises like light running, swimming, or cycling into rest days to advance blood stream and muscle unwinding.

Practice froth rolling or self-myofascial discharge strategies to diminish muscle pressure and further develop portability.

Pay attention to your body and change your preparation timetable to incorporate satisfactory rest days and deload weeks.

5.4 Sustenance and Hydration

Consume a decent eating regimen wealthy in supplements, including macronutrients (proteins, sugars, fats) and micronutrients (nutrients and minerals).

Remain hydrated by drinking a sufficient measure of water over the course of the day, and think about electrolyte renewal during extraordinary active work.

Refuel with a post-exercise feast or tidbit that incorporates protein and carbs to help muscle fix and glycogen recharging.

6. The Job of Expert Direction

6.1 Medical services Suppliers

In the event that you battle with ongoing weariness, rest unsettling influences, or tireless pressure, consider talking with a medical care supplier. They can assess your physical and psychological wellness, give direction, and suggest medicines or intercessions on a case by case basis.

6.2 Mentors and Coaches

Competitors and people associated with organized preparing projects can profit from the skill of mentors and coaches. These experts can configuration preparing plans that incorporate fitting rest and recuperation periods, assisting people with accomplishing their exhibition objectives securely and actually.

7.2 Sleep and Muscular Strength

Rest is a key part of human physiology, and its importance stretches out a long ways past the domain of rest and revival. It assumes a significant part in different physical processes, including the turn of events and support of strong strength. In this investigation, we will dive into the unpredictable connection among rest and strong strength, revealing how the amount and nature of rest can impact a person's actual exhibition and generally wellbeing.

1. **Figuring out Solid Strength**

   1.1 Meaning of Strong Strength

   Strong strength alludes to the most extreme power that muscles can produce during a solitary constriction. It is a critical part of actual wellness and assumes a fundamental part in ordinary exercises and athletic execution. Strong strength is regularly estimated through practices like weightlifting, where people lift logically heavier loads to evaluate their solidarity levels.

   1.2 Significance of Strong Strength

   Useful Development: Ordinary undertakings, for example, lifting, conveying, and pushing depend on solid strength.

   Sports Execution: Strength is a foundation of athletic achievement, adding to power, speed, and perseverance.

   Injury Avoidance: Solid muscles assist with balancing out joints and decrease the gamble of wounds.

   By and large Wellbeing: Solid strength is related with worked on metabolic wellbeing and diminished hazard of persistent illnesses.

2. **Rest Design**

   2.1 Rest Stages

   Rest is a perplexing cycle that happens in unmistakable stages, essentially partitioned into two classes: non-quick eye development

(NREM) and fast eye development (REM) rest.

NREM Rest: Containing three phases (N1, N2, and N3), NREM rest is portrayed by extending unwinding and diminishing mindfulness.

REM Rest: REM rest is the stage related with clear dreams, fast eye development, and expanded cerebrum movement.

These rest stages cycle over the course of the evening, with each stage serving explicit capabilities in physical and mental reclamation.

2.2 Rest Cycles

A total rest cycle endures roughly an hour and a half and incorporates both NREM and REM rest stages. Throughout the span of a night's rest, people normally experience a few cycles, with the extent of REM rest expanding as the night advances.

3. Rest and Muscle Recuperation

3.1 Muscle Fix and Development

During profound rest stages, particularly N3 (otherwise called sluggish wave rest), the body focuses on actual reclamation. This is when muscle fix and development happen. Chemicals, for example, development chemical and testosterone are delivered during profound rest, invigorating protein combination and muscle recuperation. The quality and amount of rest straightforwardly influence this cycle.

3.2 Glycogen Renewal

Rest likewise assumes a part in renewing glycogen stores in muscles and the liver. Glycogen is the essential energy hotspot for extreme focus exercises, and its reclamation is critical for ideal execution. Quality rest guarantees proficient glycogen renewal.

4. The Effect of Rest on Strong Strength

4.1 Hormonal Equilibrium

Chemicals assume a critical part in solid strength improvement. Development chemical and testosterone, the two of which are impacted by rest, add to muscle fix, protein combination, and generally strength. Upset or deficient rest can prompt hormonal uneven characters, possibly thwarting strength gains.

4.2 Recuperation and Muscle Irritation

Sufficient rest upholds viable recuperation by decreasing muscle touchiness and irritation. At the point when people experience lack of sleep, they are bound to feel irritation and inconvenience after serious exercises. This can affect their capacity to prepare reliably and gain ground in developing fortitude.

4.3 Muscle Coordination and Execution

Rest likewise influences muscle coordination and execution. Absence of rest can hinder neuromuscular capability, prompting diminished coordinated abilities, more slow response times, and compromised coordination. Competitors and strength coaches might find it trying to perform at their best when restless.

5. The Rest Strong Strength Association

5.1 Rest Amount

The suggested measure of rest for grown-ups normally falls between 7-9 hours out of each evening. Accomplishing this amount of rest reliably is fundamental for supporting strong strength advancement and upkeep. Lack of sleep, characterized as reliably getting under 7 hours of rest, can adversely affect strength gains.

5.2 Rest Quality

Rest quality is similarly indispensable as rest amount. People who experience regular enlightenments, rest aggravations, or rest issues may not benefit completely from their time spent in bed. Quality rest includes continuous, profound rest cycles that take into account compelling strong recuperation and chemical guideline.

5.3 Rest Consistency

Consistency in rest designs, including heading to sleep and awakening simultaneously every day, manages the body's inside clock. Unpredictable rest designs or incessant interruptions can upset circadian rhythms, possibly influencing hormonal equilibrium and by and large wellbeing.

6. Reasonable Techniques for Further developing Rest and Solid Strength

6.1 Focus on Rest Cleanliness

Keep a steady rest plan by hitting the sack and awakening simultaneously day to day.

Establish an agreeable rest climate with a steady sleeping pad, suitable room temperature, and negligible light and commotion.

Try not to animate exercises before sleep time, for example, screen time or extraordinary activity.

Limit caffeine and liquor consumption, particularly in the hours paving the way to rest.

Practice unwinding strategies like profound breathing or contemplation to quiet the psyche before rest.

6.2 Oversee Pressure

Constant pressure can disturb rest designs and hormonal equilibrium. Consolidating pressure the board strategies, like care, yoga, or moderate muscle unwinding, can assist with decreasing feelings of anxiety and further develop rest quality.

6.3 Nourishment and Exercise

Consume a fair eating routine wealthy in supplements, including macronutrients (proteins, starches, fats) and micronutrients (nutrients and minerals).

Remain hydrated by drinking a sufficient measure of water over the course of the day, and think about electrolyte renewal during extraordinary active work.

Participate in customary activity, however stay away from overwhelming exercises near sleep time, as they can be animating and disturb rest.

6.4 Look for Proficient Direction

People encountering constant rest unsettling influences or looking for customized direction for strength preparing ought to consider talking with medical care suppliers or guaranteed wellness experts. These specialists can give custom-made proposals and mediations.

7.3 Stretching, Mobility, and Foam Rolling

Extending, versatility activities, and froth rolling are fundamental parts of a balanced wellness and wellbeing schedule. These practices add to further developed adaptability,

joint wellbeing, and generally speaking actual execution. In this complete investigation, we will dig into the meaning of extending, versatility work, and froth rolling, their singular advantages, and how to integrate them into your day to day wellness routine.

1. **Extending**

   1.1 Figuring out Extending

   Extending is the act of purposefully stretching and lengthening muscles to further develop adaptability and scope of movement. It tends to be proceeded as an independent movement or as a feature of a warm-up or chill off everyday practice previously or after work out. There are different sorts of extending, including static extending, dynamic extending, and proprioceptive neuro-muscular assistance (PNF) extending.

   1.2 Advantages of Extending

   Further developed Adaptability: Standard extending can build the scope of movement in joints and muscles, considering greater developments.

   Improved Muscle Length: Extending keeps up with or increment muscle length, lessening the gamble of muscle uneven characters and injury.

   Diminished Muscle Pressure: Extending can alleviate muscle snugness and inconvenience, advancing unwinding and stress decrease.

   Further developed Stance: Extending practices that target explicit muscle gatherings can support rectifying postural irregular characteristics.

2. **Versatility Activities**

2.1 Meaning of Versatility

Versatility alludes to a singular's capacity to move joints and muscles openly through their full scope of movement. Dissimilar to adaptability, which centers around muscle protracting, portability envelops joint wellbeing, steadiness, and the capacity to productively move. Portability practices are intended to work on joint capability and upgrade generally development quality.

2.2 Advantages of Portability Activities

Joint Wellbeing: Portability practices support joint wellbeing by keeping up with synovial liquid, decreasing mileage, and forestalling firmness.

Injury Anticipation: Further developed joint portability can diminish the gamble of abuse wounds, like tendonitis or joint impingements.

Utilitarian Development: Improved versatility considers more productive and powerful practical developments in day to day existence and sports exercises.

Further developed Execution: Competitors can profit from expanded portability as it improves readiness, speed, and coordination.

3. **Froth Rolling**

3.1 Froth Rolling Characterized

Froth rolling, otherwise called self-myofascial discharge, is a self-knead method that includes utilizing a froth roller to apply strain to explicit muscle gatherings. The objective is to deliver pressure and bonds inside the sash, a connective tissue that encompasses muscles. Froth rolling is frequently performed previously or after exercise to further develop muscle capability and diminish muscle irritation.

3.2 Advantages of Froth Rolling

Myofascial Delivery: Froth moving aides discharge bunches and attachments in the belt, which can alleviate muscle snugness and further develop portability.

Muscle Recuperation: Utilizing a froth roller after exercise can diminish muscle irritation and work with quicker recuperation.

Injury Counteraction: Normal froth rolling can assist with forestalling abuse wounds by tending to muscle lopsided characteristics and diminishing strain.

Further developed Scope of Movement: Froth rolling can upgrade joint versatility and work on the scope of movement in designated muscle gatherings.

4. **Integrating Extending, Portability, and Froth Moving into Your Daily practice**

4.1 Warm-Up and Chill Off

Warm-Up: Powerful extending and versatility practices are great for setting up your muscles and joints for more extraordinary actual work. Center around developments that impersonate the activities you intend to perform.

Cool-Down: After work out, perform static extending and froth moving to loosen up muscles, discharge pressure, and advance recuperation.

4.2 Day to day Portability Practice

Integrate day to day portability practices into your daily schedule to improve in general joint wellbeing and development quality. Focus on key regions like the hips, shoulders, and spine, as these locales frequently benefit the most from versatility work.

4.3 Designated Froth Rolling

Utilize a froth roller to target explicit muscle bunches that might be tight or sore. Roll gradually over the muscle, applying moderate tension. On the off chance that you experience an especially weakness, stop and inhale profoundly to assist with delivering strain.

4.4 Extending Schedule

Plan an extending schedule that tends to your singular requirements and objectives. Incorporate both static and dynamic stretches for a balanced practice. Center around extending the significant muscle gatherings of the body, like the hamstrings, quadriceps, hip flexors, chest, and back.

5. **Normal Mix-ups and Precautionary measures**

5.1 Overextending

Abstain from overextending, as it can prompt muscle strains or wounds. Stretch inside your scope of movement and never force a stretch. A delicate and steady methodology is more compelling and more secure over the long haul.

5.2 Skipping

Try not to skip or utilize snapping developments while extending. This can cause miniature tears in the muscle filaments and increment the gamble of injury. All things considered, hold each stretch for 15-30 seconds and inhale profoundly to unwind into it.

5.3 Froth Moving Torment

While some inconvenience during froth rolling is ordinary, it ought not be horrifying. On the off chance that you experience extreme torment, pause and counsel a medical care proficient. Froth rolling shouldn't cause injury or deteriorate existing circumstances.

5.4 Prior Wounds

On the off chance that you have previous wounds or ailments, talk with a medical services supplier or actual specialist prior to starting an extending, versatility, or froth moving daily schedule. They can give customized direction and changes.

Chapter 8

Assessing and Tracking Muscular Strength

Strong strength is a central part of actual wellness and assumes a critical part in everyday exercises, sports execution, and generally speaking prosperity. Evaluating and following solid strength is fundamental for people hoping to further develop their solidarity levels, improve their preparation projects, and screen their advancement over the long run. In this thorough aide, we will dig into the different strategies and procedures used to evaluate and follow strong strength, the significance of doing as such, and how to actually decipher and apply the outcomes.

1. **Grasping Strong Strength**
   1.1 Meaning of Solid Strength
   Solid strength is the capacity of a muscle or gathering of muscles to produce force against opposition. It is regularly estimated in units of power, like pounds or kilograms, and is well defined for specific developments or activities. Solid strength is fundamental for different exercises, including lifting, pushing, pulling, and conveying, and it adds to sports execution, injury avoidance, and everyday practical assignments.
   1.2 Significance of Strong Strength

Sports Execution: In many games, including weightlifting, powerlifting, and running, solid strength straightforwardly corresponds with progress and upper hand.

Injury Counteraction: Solid muscles assist with settling joints and lessen the gamble of wounds, particularly in exercises that include influence or unexpected developments.

Utilitarian Errands: Everyday exercises like climbing steps, lifting food, or moving furniture require strong strength.

Metabolic Wellbeing: Solid strength is related with worked on metabolic wellbeing, including better insulin responsiveness and metabolic rate.

2. **Strategies for Evaluating Strong Strength**

2.1 One-Rep Max (1RM) Testing

Practice Determination: Pick practices that focus on the particular muscle gathering or development design you need to survey (e.g., seat press for chest strength).

Warm-Up: Preceding 1RM testing, play out an exhaustive get ready to forestall injury and set up the muscles for maximal exertion.

Moderate Stacking: Begin with a light weight and bit by bit increment the heap until the individual can at this point unfinished a solitary redundancy with legitimate structure.

2.2 Redundancy Most extreme (RM) Testing

3RM: The most extreme weight an individual can lift for three reiterations.

5RM: The most extreme weight an individual can lift for five reiterations.

10RM: The greatest weight an individual can lift for ten reiterations.

2.3 Isometric Testing

Isometric testing includes evaluating solid strength by estimating the power created when a muscle contracts against an undaunted item or obstruction. While more uncommon than dynamic strength testing, isometric evaluations can be important for explicit applications, like restoration or injury avoidance.

2.4 Handheld Dynamometers

Handheld dynamometers are convenient gadgets used to quantify the power applied by unambiguous muscle gatherings. They are regularly utilized in clinical settings and give quantitative information to surveying muscle strength in people with wounds or ailments.

2.5 Useful Strength Testing

Useful strength tests assess a singular's capacity to carry out unambiguous practical developments that require strength and security. Models incorporate the squat, deadlift, or rancher's walk. Useful strength testing surveys how well a singular's solidarity converts into commonsense, certifiable developments.

3. Following Solid Strength

3.1 The Significance of Following

Objective Setting: Following permits people to set explicit, quantifiable, and attainable strength-related objectives.

Program Advancement: Checking progress changes preparing projects to guarantee proceeded with progress and forestall levels.

Inspiration: Following advancement can be exceptionally spurring, giving uplifting feedback to difficult work and commitment.

Injury Avoidance: Recognizing critical strength awkward nature or declines can act as an early advance notice indication of likely injury.

3.2 Recurrence of Appraisal

Occasional Evaluation: Lead appraisals at normal stretches, like each 4 two months, to check progress and change preparing plans.

Persistent Checking: A few competitors and mentors ceaselessly track strength by recording each instructional course's presentation.

4. Apparatuses and Methods for Following Strong Strength

4.1 Preparation Logs

Preparing logs or diaries are straightforward yet viable instruments for following strength gains. People record subtleties of every exercise, including works out, sets, reiterations, and the weight lifted. Preparing logs can be actual note pads or advanced applications intended for wellness following.

4.2 Moderate Over-burden

Moderate over-burden is an essential rule of solidarity preparing that includes progressively expanding the obstruction or force of activities over the long haul. By reliably testing muscles with heavier loads or more noteworthy opposition, people can follow strength gains.

4.3 Redundancy and Burden Movement

In RM testing, following the quantity of reiterations performed at a given weight gives significant information. Over the long run, as people can perform more reiterations at a specific weight, it shows an expansion in solid perseverance and, in a roundabout way, strength.

4.4 Mechanical Apparatuses

Progressions in wellness innovation have presented different apparatuses and gadgets for following strong strength:

Wearable Wellness Trackers: Numerous wearable wellness gadgets can track and record exercise information, including reiterations, sets, and burden lifted.

Strength Following Applications: There are various cell phone applications planned explicitly for strength following, giving elements, for example, exercise logging and progress charts.

Electronic Strength Testing Gadgets: Some high level exercise center hardware comes outfitted with electronic frameworks that track and show strength measurements, gaining it simple to screen headway.

5. Deciphering and Applying Strength Appraisal Results

5.1 Defining Reasonable Objectives

Deciphering appraisal results is the most vital phase in setting reasonable and feasible strength-related objectives. Whether the objective is to increment 1RM, further develop perseverance, or upgrade practical strength, the evaluation information gives a benchmark from which to work.

5.2 Program Change

Consistently following strong strength takes into consideration informed program changes. On the off chance that progress slows down or declines, mentors and people can alter preparing factors like activity choice, volume, power, or recurrence to get through levels and move along.

5.3 Distinguishing Shortcomings and Lopsided characteristics

Strength evaluations can uncover shortcomings or lopsided characteristics in unambiguous muscle gatherings or development designs. Tending to these shortcomings through designated activities and restorative techniques can improve by and large strength and diminish the gamble of injury.

5.4 Observing Injury Recuperation

For people recuperating from wounds, it is urgent to follow solid strength. It helps check recovery progress and guarantees that strength levels return to pre-injury levels prior to continuing normal preparation.

6. Wellbeing Contemplations and Precautionary measures

6.1 Appropriate Procedure

Keeping up with appropriate procedure during strength appraisals is vital to guarantee precise outcomes and forestall injury. Lift loads with legitimate structure, and look for direction from a certified mentor or mentor if necessary.

6.2 Moderate Over-burden

While it's crucial for challenge muscles logically, stay away from unreasonably significant burdens or unexpected expansions in opposition, as this can prompt wounds, including strains or injuries.

6.3 Recuperation

Satisfactory rest and recuperation are imperative to forestall overtraining and advance strength gains. Muscles expect time to fix and adjust to expanded loads. Integrate rest days into your preparation program.

6.4 Expert Direction

People with explicit objectives or complex preparation needs, like competitors or those with ailments, may profit from working with confirmed strength and molding trained professionals or actual specialists who can give customized evaluations and direction.

8.1 Measuring Strength (1RM and Isometric Testing)

Strength is a central part of actual wellness and assumes a pivotal part in different parts of life, from everyday exercises to sports execution. Estimating strength is fundamental for competitors, wellness devotees, and medical care experts to survey a singular's capacities, screen progress, and designer preparing or restoration programs likewise. In this far reaching guide, we will dig into two critical techniques for estimating strength: One-Rep Most extreme (1RM) testing and isometric testing. We will investigate their standards, applications, benefits, and how they add to advancing execution and wellbeing.

1. **Figuring out Strength Estimation**
   1.1 Meaning of Solidarity
   Strength alludes to the limit of muscles or muscle gatherings to produce force against opposition. It is commonly evaluated in units of power, like pounds or kilograms. Strength estimation permits us to decide a singular's most extreme power yield and evaluate their capacity to perform errands that require beating opposition, for example, lifting loads, moving items, or keeping up with act.

1.2 Significance of Solidarity Estimation

Execution Assessment: Strength appraisals assist competitors with measuring their abilities and put forth execution objectives.

Preparing Solution: Wellness experts use strength estimations to plan compelling preparation programs custom-made to a singular's capacities and goals.

Restoration: Strength testing is important in injury recovery to screen progress and decide when an individual is prepared to get back to standard exercises.

Following Advancement: Ordinary strength estimation permits people to screen their preparation headway and make vital changes.

2. **One-Rep Greatest (1RM) Testing**

2.1 What is 1RM Trying?

One-Rep Greatest (1RM) testing is a generally utilized strategy to survey a person's maximal strength for a particular activity. It includes deciding the most extreme weight an individual can lift for a solitary reiteration with legitimate structure. 1RM testing is frequently utilized for compound activities like the squat, seat press, or deadlift.

2.2 Standards of 1RM Testing

Practice Determination: Pick an activity that objectives the muscle gathering or development example of interest.

Warm-Up: Play out an exhaustive get ready to set up the muscles and joints for maximal exertion and decrease the gamble of injury.

Moderate Stacking: Begin with a generally light weight and continuously increment the heap until the individual can at this point unfinished a solitary reiteration with legitimate structure.

2.3 Utilizations of 1RM Testing

1RM testing has different applications:

Strength Evaluation: It gives a pattern estimation of a person's maximal strength.

Program Plan: Wellness experts utilize 1RM information to tailor strength preparing programs by deciding proper opposition levels and exercise determination.

Checking Progress: Consistently retesting 1RM permits people to follow their solidarity gains and change their preparation in like manner.

2.4 Benefits of 1RM Testing

1RM testing offers a few benefits:

Objective Estimation: It gives an unmistakable and objective estimation of a person's maximal strength.

Individualization: 1RM testing considers customized preparing programs in light of a singular's particular abilities.

Inspiration: Accomplishing new 1RM achievements can be profoundly rousing and support the advantages of reliable preparation.

3. Isometric Testing

3.1 What is Isometric Trying?

Isometric testing includes evaluating strong strength by estimating the power produced when a muscle contracts against an unflinching item or opposition. Not at all like unique developments in 1RM testing, isometric testing includes static compressions where the muscle length doesn't change. Isometric testing can be utilized to survey explicit muscle gatherings or joint solidness.

3.2 Standards of Isometric Testing

Situating: People keep a particular joint point or stance while applying maximal power against a resolute item or opposition.

Steadiness: The article or obstruction ought to be steady and relentless to precisely gauge the power produced.

Recording Power: Particular gear, for example, handheld dynamometers or power plates, is frequently used to evaluate the power applied during the isometric withdrawal.

3.3 Uses of Isometric Testing

Muscle Detachment: It takes into consideration the appraisal of explicit muscle gatherings or segregated joint dependability.

Restoration: Isometric testing is important in non-intrusive treatment to survey and screen muscle strength during the recuperation cycle.

Practical Testing: Isometric tests can mirror utilitarian developments and survey a

singular's capacity to keep up with security in different positions.

3.4 Benefits of Isometric Testing

Security: Isometric testing is by and large more secure than dynamic developments, as there is no joint development included.

Muscle Separation: It empowers the appraisal of individual muscle gatherings, making it appropriate for distinguishing muscle uneven characters.

Reproducibility: Isometric tests are profoundly reproducible, taking into consideration predictable and precise estimations over the long haul.

4. Looking at 1RM and Isometric Testing

4.1 Particularity of Estimation

1RM testing basically surveys a person's maximal strength for dynamic developments, for example, lifting loads. Interestingly, isometric testing can assess static strength and joint soundness, giving an alternate point of view on a singular's capacities.

4.2 Security and Chance

1RM testing can represent a higher gamble of injury, especially when people endeavor maximal lifts. Isometric testing, then again, is for the most part more secure as it doesn't include dynamic developments or weighty burdens.

4.3 Hardware Necessities

1RM testing regularly expects admittance to explicit obstruction gear, like free weights, free weights, or weight machines. Isometric testing might require particular gear, for example, handheld dynamometers or power plates.

4.4 Appropriateness for Recovery

Isometric testing is many times liked in recovery settings, where patients might have restrictions in scope of movement or dynamic development. Isometric tests can help survey and screen progress without intensifying existing wounds.

5. **Directing 1RM and Isometric Testing**

5.1 Pre-Testing Contemplations

Wellbeing Screening: Guarantee that people are actually equipped for taking part in strength testing and have no hidden ailments that contraindicate testing.

Warm-Up: Incorporate a far reaching warm-up daily practice to set up the muscles and joints for maximal exertion.

Security Measures: Execute wellbeing measures, like spotters for 1RM testing and legitimate hardware arrangement for isometric testing.

5.2 1RM Testing Convention

Practice Determination: Pick a proper activity for the muscle gathering or development design you need to evaluate.

Warm-Up Sets: Perform warm-up sets with dynamically heavier loads to set up the muscles and sensory system for maximal exertion.

Maximal Endeavor: Play out a maximal endeavor, step by step expanding the load until the individual can presently unfinished a solitary reiteration with legitimate structure.

5.3 Isometric Testing Convention

Situating: Set up the person in the ideal position, keeping up with the joint point or stance you need to survey.

Adjustment: Guarantee that the item or obstruction utilized for the isometric constriction is steady and secure.

Recording Power: Utilize specific hardware to gauge and record the power created during the isometric compression.

6. **Deciphering Results and Applications**

6.1 Deciphering 1RM Outcomes

Benchmark Appraisal: Decide the singular's pattern strength level for the particular activity.

Objective Setting: Utilize 1RM information to set practical and attainable strength-related objectives.

Program Configuration: Plan strength preparing programs custom-made to the person's 1RM abilities and targets.

6.2 Deciphering Isometric Outcomes

Muscle Evaluation: Recognize muscle lopsided characteristics or shortcomings in unambiguous muscle gatherings or joint soundness.

Recovery Observing: Screen muscle strength during restoration to evaluate progress and status for return to ordinary exercises.

Utilitarian Assessment: Evaluate a singular's capacity to keep up with strength in different positions or during explicit practical developments.

6.3 Strength Preparing Applications

1RM-Based Projects: Utilize 1RM information to recommend obstruction levels for strength preparing activities and track progress.

Isometric Activities: Integrate isometric activities into preparing projects to address explicit shortcomings or work on joint steadiness.

Recovery: Use isometric testing to plan and screen restoration programs for people recuperating from wounds.

8.2 Functional Assessments

Useful evaluation is a basic part of actual wellbeing assessment that spotlights on a singular's capacity to perform ordinary developments and exercises successfully and without torment. This appraisal distinguishes impediments, lopsided characteristics, or dysfunctions in the outer muscle and neuromuscular frameworks, helping with the advancement of customized restoration or work out schedules. In this extensive aide, we will dive into the standards, procedures, and utilizations of utilitarian appraisal, underlining its significance in advancing ideal development and generally prosperity.

1. **Grasping Useful Appraisal**
   1.1 Meaning of Useful Evaluation
   Useful appraisal is the most common way of assessing a singular's development designs, joint portability, muscle strength, adaptability, solidness, and neuromuscular control to decide their capacity to carry out practical exercises. These exercises might incorporate strolling, running, crouching, lifting, coming to, from there, the sky is the limit. Useful evaluation goes past disengaged joint or muscle assessments and thinks about how various parts cooperate during complex developments.
   1.2 Significance of Useful Appraisal
   Recognizing Dysfunctions: It distinguishes development dysfunctions, uneven characters, or constraints that might prompt torment, injury, or diminished execution.

   Fitting Intercessions: Results from practical appraisals guide the improvement of customized recovery or work out schedules that address explicit impediments and upgrade generally speaking capability.

   Checking Progress: Standard useful evaluations permit people and experts to follow enhancements, change mediations, and forestall likely misfortunes.

   Injury Counteraction: By recognizing and tending to development dysfunctions, useful appraisal can lessen the gamble of future wounds or abuse conditions.

2. **Standards of Useful Evaluation**
   2.1 Development Examples
   Crouching: Surveying the capacity to play out a legitimate squat, which is principal for some exercises.
   Lurching: Assessing single-leg rushing developments to check for equilibrium and security.
   Coming to: Surveying chest area versatility and steadiness during arriving at
   developments.

Strolling and Running: Dissecting stride designs for any deviations or anomalies.

Practical Errands: Assessing the capacity to carry out unambiguous useful undertakings, for example, lifting articles or climbing steps.

2.2 Joint Portability

Surveying joint portability includes assessing the scope of movement (ROM) in different joints, including the spine, hips, knees, and shoulders. Limited joint portability can influence development effectiveness and lead to pay or lopsided characteristics.

2.3 Muscle Strength

Muscle strength evaluation includes testing the strength of explicit muscle bunches utilizing different procedures, for example, manual muscle testing, obstruction activities,

or isometric constrictions. Muscle awkward nature or shortcomings can add to unfortunate development examples and increment the gamble of injury.

2.4 Adaptability and Scope of Movement

Adaptability evaluations center around a singular's capacity to move joints through their full scope of movement without inconvenience or restrictions. Limited adaptability can obstruct practical developments and lead to compensatory designs.

2.5 Dependability and Neuromuscular Control

Dependability and neuromuscular control appraisals assess a singular's capacity to control and balance out their body during developments and utilitarian errands. Unfortunate soundness can prompt wasteful developments and an expanded gamble of falls or wounds.

3. Strategies for Useful Evaluation

3.1 Development Screens

Development screens include a progression of explicit developments or errands that people perform under perception. One notable model is the Useful Development Screen (FMS), which evaluates key development examples, portability, and strength.

3.2 Joint Evaluation

Joint appraisals include assessing the scope of movement (ROM) in individual joints utilizing normalized estimations or useful tests. These evaluations might incorporate goniometry or joint-explicit tests like the Thomas test for hip flexor snugness.

3.3 Muscle Strength Testing

Muscle strength testing can be led utilizing different strategies, for example, manual muscle testing, handheld dynamometers, or opposition works out. These tests survey muscle gatherings' solidarity and recognize shortcomings or awkward nature.

3.4 Adaptability Tests

Adaptability tests measure a singular's scope of movement in un-ambiguous joints or muscle gatherings. Models incorporate the sit-and-arrive at test for hamstring adaptability or the shoulder flexion test for chest area portability.

3.5 Equilibrium and Dependability Appraisals

Equilibrium and dependability appraisals incorporate single-leg balance tests, proprioceptive activities, and useful undertakings that challenge a singular's capacity to control their body during dynamic developments.

4. Practical Evaluation Applications

4.1 Injury Recovery

Useful evaluations are vital in injury restoration. They assist medical care experts with distinguishing development dysfunctions or muscle lopsided characteristics that might have added to the injury. Recovery projects can then be customized to resolve these issues, advance mending, and forestall re-injury.

4.2 Prehabilitation

Prehabilitation includes addressing development restrictions and uneven characters before they lead to wounds. Practical evaluations can recognize possible issues, permitting people to pro-actively work on further developing their development examples and decreasing injury risk.

4.3 Games Execution Upgrade

Useful evaluations are important for competitors looking to advance their presentation. By recognizing shortcomings or constraints in development and capability, competitors can consolidate designated activities and preparing techniques to upgrade their athletic capacities.

4.4 General Wellness

Utilitarian evaluations are not restricted to competitors or people with wounds. They are significant for anyone with any interest in working on their wellness and in general prosperity. By tending to development limits and uneven characters, people can upgrade their everyday exercises and lessen the gamble of agony or injury.

5. Deciphering Useful Evaluation Results

5.1 Distinguishing Impediments and Dysfunctions

Deciphering useful evaluation results includes recognizing explicit constraints, dysfunctions, or awkward nature in a singular's development designs, joint portability, muscle strength, adaptability, soundness, or neuromuscular control.

5.2 Putting forth Objectives

In view of the evaluation discoveries, people and experts can set explicit, quantifiable, attainable, important, and time-bound (Brilliant) objectives for further developing development and capability.

5.3 Fitting Intercessions

The consequences of useful appraisals guide the improvement of custom-made intercessions, including exercise programs, portability drills, steadiness works out, and

neuromuscular preparation, pointed toward tending to distinguished impediments or lopsided characteristics.

5.4 Following Advancement

Normal reassessment of useful boundaries permits people and experts to follow progress, make essential changes in accordance with mediations, and guarantee that objectives are being met.

8.3 Effective Tracking Techniques

Powerful following strategies are significant devices for people endeavoring to improve efficiency, accomplish objectives, and keep up with coordinated and organized lives. Following includes deliberately recording and observing different parts of one's life, undertakings, or progress toward explicit goals. In this far reaching guide, we will investigate the standards and advantages of viable following procedures, talk about different areas where following is useful, and give down to earth experiences and techniques to effective following.

1. **Grasping Successful Following Methods**

   1.1 Meaning of Following

   Following includes the consistent assortment and recording of information or data connected with explicit exercises, assignments, objectives, or propensities. It assists people with acquiring experiences, measure headway, and pursue educated choices in different viewpoints regarding their own and proficient lives.

   1.2 Significance of Powerful Following

   Upgraded Efficiency: Following assists people with remaining coordinated, focus on undertakings, and dispense time and assets effectively.

   Objective Accomplishment: It empowers people to define clear objectives, screen headway, and make vital changes in accordance with keep focused.

   Information Driven Choices: Following gives information and bits of knowledge that illuminate choices, permitting people to settle on informed decisions and advance results.

   Responsibility: Standard following advances responsibility by considering people liable for their activities and progress.

2. Standards of Compelling Following

2.1 Lucidity of Targets

Obviously characterized targets are essential to successful following. Whether following undertakings, objectives, propensities, or costs, knowing definitively what you plan to accomplish gives major areas of strength for a to the following system.

2.2 Consistency

Consistency in following is critical to acquiring significant information. Lay out a customary timetable and routine for following exercises, and stick to it tirelessly. Consistency guarantees that information is extensive and dependable.

2.3 Quantifiable Measurements

Pick measurements or boundaries that are quantifiable and applicable to your targets. For instance, if following individual budgets, consider measurements like pay, costs, reserve funds, and obligation decrease.

2.4 Information Assortment

Utilize dependable strategies and apparatuses for information assortment. This might include manual keep in journals or advanced following through applications and programming. Guarantee the information assortment process is helpful and available.

2.5 Examination and Reflection

Following isn't just about recording information; it additionally includes breaking down and considering the data assembled. Routinely survey your following information to recognize examples, patterns, and regions for development.

3. Spaces of Viable Following

3.1 Using time productively

Following time is pivotal for powerful using time productively. Procedures like time logs, Pomodoro following, and time-impeding can assist people with understanding how they dispense their time and make fundamental changes for more prominent efficiency.

3.2 Assignment and Task The board

Following errands and undertakings guarantees that people stay coordinated and fulfill time constraints. Daily agendas, project the executives programming, and assignment following applications are significant devices in this space.

3.3 Monetary Administration

Following individual budgets includes checking pay, costs, reserve funds, ventures, and obligation. Planning applications and monetary accounting sheets are ordinarily utilized for monetary following.

3.4 Wellbeing and Health

Following wellbeing and health information, for example, diet, work out, rest designs, and imperative measurements, enables people to settle on informed conclusions about their prosperity. Wellbeing applications, wellness trackers, and journaling are normal strategies for wellbeing following.

3.5 Objective Accomplishment

Following advancement toward objectives is fundamental for accomplishing them. People can utilize objective following applications, diaries, or objective explicit measurements to screen their headway and make important changes.

4. Viable Following Methods

4.1 Savvy Objectives

Take on the Shrewd (Explicit, Quantifiable, Attainable, Pertinent, Time-bound) structure while putting forth objectives. Savvy objectives give clear rules to following advancement and estimating achievement.

4.2 Assignment Records and Prioritization

Make day to day or week after week task records and focus on them in view of significance and criticalness. Apparatuses like Eisenhower's Earnest/Significant Grid can support task prioritization.

4.3 Propensity Following

Creating positive propensities is attainable through propensity following. Reliably record the day to day or week after week pursue of wanted routines, and use propensity following applications or diaries to imagine progress.

4.4 Time Logs

Time logs include recording how time is gone through over the course of the day. Breaking down time logs assists people with distinguishing time-burning through exercises and apportion time all the more really.

4.5 Journaling and Intelligent Composition

Keeping a diary or journal permits people to follow individual encounters, contemplations, and feelings. Intelligent composing can give experiences into ways of behaving and profound prosperity.

4.6 Monetary Following Devices

Different monetary following devices are accessible, including planning applications, cost trackers, and speculation portfolio chiefs. These devices improve on monetary following and give experiences into ways of managing money.

4.7 Undertaking The executives Programming

For complex activities, project the board programming like Trello, Asana, or Microsoft Task offers powerful following abilities. They empower joint effort, task, and undertaking progress observing.

4.8 Computerized Schedules

Advanced schedules, for example, Google Schedule or Microsoft Viewpoint are superb for following arrangements, cutoff times, and occasions. They offer updates and warnings to assist people with remaining coordinated.

5. Advantages of Compelling Following

5.1 Upgraded Efficiency

Following empowers people to distinguish time-squandering exercises, enhance time portion, and spotlight on high-need undertakings, bringing about expanded efficiency.

5.2 Objective Accomplishment

Viable following guarantees people stay on track toward their objectives. It gives an internal compass, measures headway, and assists them with settling on informed choices to accomplish their targets.

5.3 Better Independent direction

Information driven direction is worked with by following. By examining information and examples, people can go with informed decisions and changes in different everyday issues.

5.4 Responsibility

Following considers people responsible for their activities and progress. At the point when they see their presentation reported, they are bound to stick to responsibilities and make upgrades.

6. Difficulties and Tips for Successful Following

6.1 Overcomplication

Stay away from overcomplicating global positioning frameworks. Keep them basic, natural, and lined up with your targets. Intricacy can prompt disappointment and diminished adherence.

6.2 Consistency

Keeping up with consistency in following can challenge. Lay out a daily schedule and set suggestions to guarantee normal information assortment.

6.3 Information Over-burden

Gathering unreasonable information can overpower. Center around key measurements that line up with your objectives to stay away from information over-burden.

6.4 Adaptability

Be adaptable in adjusting following strategies and devices on a case by case basis. What works today might require changes tomorrow founded on changing conditions or objectives.

Chapter 9

Injury Prevention, Rehabilitation, and Real-World Applications

Injury counteraction and restoration are basic parts of keeping up with actual wellbeing and prosperity, whether you're a competitor, a functioning individual, or just somebody hoping to carry on with a better life. This extensive aide investigates the standards and procedures of injury anticipation, the restoration cycle, and certifiable utilizations of these ideas. By understanding how to forestall wounds, explore the recovery venture, and apply these standards in day to day existence, people can lead better, more dynamic, and without injury lives.

1. **Injury Anticipation**
   1.1 Meaning of Injury Anticipation
   Injury counteraction alludes to a proactive methodology pointed toward diminishing the gamble of wounds before they happen. It includes a great many methodologies and measures intended to advance security and limit the potential for mishaps or actual mischief.
   1.2 Significance of Injury Avoidance
   Improved Personal satisfaction: Forestalling wounds jelly actual

wellbeing, versatility, and by and large prosperity, empowering people to partake in a functioning and satisfying life.

Diminished Medical care Expenses: Less wounds mean decreased medical care costs, both for people and the medical care framework.

Further developed Efficiency: Wounds frequently bring about time off work or decreased efficiency. Forestalling wounds benefits people and managers the same.

Long haul Prosperity: Powerful injury counteraction measures can significantly affect long haul wellbeing, diminishing the gamble of persistent torment and unexpected problems.

2. **Methodologies for Injury Avoidance**

2.1 Practical preparation

Functional preparing includes standard activity and strength preparing to further develop muscle strength, adaptability, and perseverance. Appropriate molding decreases the gamble of abuse wounds and improves by and large actual versatility.

2.2 Appropriate Procedure

Utilizing appropriate strategy during proactive tasks and activities is fundamental. Preparing with right structure limits the gamble of intense wounds brought about by ill-advised developments and biomechanical stress.

2.3 Warm-Up and Chill Off

Warm-up schedules set up the body for practice by expanding blood stream and adaptability. Chilling off after action supports muscle recuperation and diminishes the gamble of post-practice wounds.

2.4 Sufficient Rest and Recuperation

Offsetting active work with rest and recuperation is vital to forestall overtraining and ongoing wounds. Give muscles time to fix and adjust between exercises.

2.5 Defensive Hardware

For sports and exercises with intrinsic dangers, the utilization of defensive stuff like protective caps, cushions, or supports can essentially diminish the gamble of injury.

2.6 Natural Mindfulness

Monitoring natural variables, like elusive surfaces, lopsided landscape, or outrageous atmospheric conditions, can assist people with keeping away from mishaps and wounds.

3. Restoration

3.1 Meaning of Restoration

Restoration is the most common way of reestablishing capability, decreasing agony, and working on personal satisfaction following a physical issue, medical procedure, or ailment. It includes non-intrusive treatment, works out, and different mediations to recover lost capacities and upgrade by and large prosperity.

3.2 Significance of Recovery

Rebuilding of Capability: Recovery assists people with recapturing lost actual capability and versatility, permitting them to continue their day to day exercises.

Torment The board: It oversees agony and inconvenience related with wounds or ailments.

Forestalling Confusions: Restoration can forestall optional inconveniences and long haul incapacity.

Emotional well-being: The course of recovery can likewise decidedly affect psychological wellness, supporting certainty and inspiration.

4. The Restoration Interaction

4.1 Appraisal and Determination

Restoration starts with an exhaustive evaluation and finding of the injury or condition. Medical care experts assess the degree of the issue, distinguish objectives, and foster a customized recovery plan.

4.2 Laying out Objectives

Laying out clear and feasible objectives is a crucial part of recovery. Objectives might incorporate further developing scope of movement, lessening torment, recovering strength, or getting back to explicit exercises.

4.3 Individualized Treatment

Recovery programs are custom fitted to the singular's requirements and objectives. Treatment might incorporate activities, manual treatment, modalities like intensity or cold treatment, and schooling on taking care of oneself.

4.4 Moderate Activities

Actual specialists frequently utilize moderate activities to challenge and fortify harmed or debilitated regions continuously. These activities assist with advancing recuperating and reestablish capability.

4.5 Observing Advancement

Standard checking of progress is fundamental during restoration. Medical services experts survey the singular's reaction to therapy, make changes on a case by case basis, and track upgrades.

4.6 Training and Taking care of oneself

Training is a critical part of restoration. People find out about their condition, appropriate body mechanics, and techniques for forestalling future wounds.

5. Genuine Applications

5.1 Games and Sports

In the domain of sports and games, injury anticipation and recovery are vital. Competitors use procedures like warm-ups, molding, and defensive stuff to decrease injury risk. In the event of injury, immediate and successful recovery is significant for getting back to contest.

5.2 Working environment Wellbeing

Working environment wounds can have serious outcomes. Businesses carry out wellbeing measures and give preparing to decrease the gamble of mishaps. Restoration programs help representatives recuperate and get back to work.

5.3 Dynamic Way of life

For people driving dynamic ways of life, injury anticipation is fundamental. Appropriate structure, molding, and recuperation methods can delay a functioning, physical issue free life.

5.4 Maturing and Old Populace

As people age, the gamble of falls and wounds increments. Fall avoidance projects and restoration for seniors are critical to keeping up with autonomy and personal satisfaction.

5.5 Engine Vehicle Mishaps

Wounds coming about because of engine vehicle mishaps can be extreme. Recovery assumes a urgent part in assisting mishap survivors with recapturing capability and versatility.

5.6 Constant Torment The board

Persistent agony conditions frequently require continuous recovery and taking care of oneself systems. People figure out how to oversee torment, further develop capability, and upgrade their general prosperity.

6. Difficulties and Tips for Compelling Injury Avoidance and Restoration

6.1 Adherence to Restoration Plans

Remaining predictable with recovery activities and treatment plans can challenge. Defining feasible objectives, looking for help from medical services suppliers, and keeping an inspirational perspective can help.

6.2 Recognizing Chance Variables

Distinguishing individual gamble factors for wounds is fundamental for anticipation. Interview with medical care experts or experts can assist with pinpointing explicit dangers and foster designated anticipation procedures.

6.3 Conquering Dread and Vulnerability

Wounds and restoration can genuinely challenge. Looking for help from medical care experts, companions, or care groups can assist people with adapting to dread and vulnerability.

6.4 Long haul Responsibility

Injury anticipation and restoration frequently require long haul responsibility. Integrating injury anticipation techniques into everyday schedules and adhering to restoration plans are critical for progress.

9.1Common Strength Training Injuries

Strength preparing is a famous and successful method for working on solid strength, perseverance, and by and large wellness. Notwithstanding, similar to any actual work, it accompanies the gamble of injury. Understanding normal strength preparing wounds, their causes, counteraction techniques, and proper treatment is fundamental for protected and compelling preparation. In this aide, we will investigate probably the most pervasive strength preparing wounds, offering bits of knowledge into their anticipation and the board.

1. **Normal Strength Preparing Wounds**
   1.1 Injuries and Strains
   Injuries and strains are among the most widely recognized strength preparing wounds. They happen when muscles, ligaments, or tendons are extended or torn past their ability. Normal areas for injuries and strains incorporate the lower back, shoulders, and knees.
   1.2 Tendinitis
   Tendinitis, otherwise called tendonitis, is the irritation of a ligament. It frequently influences regions like the shoulders (rotator sleeve tendinitis) or elbows (tennis elbow or golf player's elbow). Tendinitis can result from dreary or abuse movements during strength preparing.
   1.3 Muscle Issues and Fits
   Muscle issues and fits include compulsory constrictions of muscles. Drying out, electrolyte uneven characters, or lacking warm-up and extending can add to issues and fits during strength preparing.
   1.4 Low Back Agony
   Low back torment is a typical grievance among strength mentors,

especially while practices including the lower back or significant burdens are involved. Unfortunate structure, inappropriate lifting methods, and muscle irregular characteristics can add to back torment.

1.5 Rotator Sleeve Wounds

Rotator sleeve wounds, like tears or strains, can happen during strength preparing practices that include above developments, similar to seat presses or shoulder presses. Powerless or imbalanced shoulder muscles might expand the gamble.

1.6 Knee Wounds

Knee wounds, including tendon injuries and meniscus tears, can happen while performing practices that include profound knee twists or abrupt course adjustments. Squats and thrusts are instances of activities that might represent a gamble.

2. Reasons for Normal Strength Preparing Wounds

2.1 Unfortunate Structure and Strategy

One of the essential drivers of solidarity preparing wounds is unfortunate structure and strategy. Utilizing erroneous structure or lifting loads that are too weighty can put inordinate weight on muscles, ligaments, and joints.

2.2 Overtraining

Overtraining happens when people participate in strength preparing too much of the time or with unnecessary volume. It can prompt exhaustion, debilitated muscles, and expanded defenselessness to wounds.

2.3 Insufficient Warm-Up and Chill Off

Skirting warm-up practices before a strength instructional meeting can make muscles more inclined to injury. Furthermore, failing to chill off appropriately can prompt muscle solidness and irritation.

2.4 Muscle Lopsided characteristics

Muscle lopsided characteristics happen when some muscle bunches are fundamentally more grounded than others. This can prompt compensatory developments and an expanded gamble of injury.

2.5 Absence of Adaptability

Lacking adaptability can restrict joint versatility and scope of movement, making it simpler to strain muscles or ligaments during strength preparing works out.

3. Counteraction of Normal Strength Preparing Wounds

3.1 Appropriate Structure and Strategy

Learning and reliably involving legitimate structure and strategy for each exercise is urgent for injury counteraction. Look for direction from a certified coach in the event that you are uncertain about your structure.

3.2 Slow Movement

Stay away from the impulse to lift significant burdens excessively fast. Progressively increment the weight and power of your activities to permit your body to securely adjust.

3.3 Sufficient Warm-Up and Chill Off

Focus on heating up with dynamic stretches and developments before your solidarity instructional course. A short time later, cool down with static stretches to keep up with adaptability and diminish muscle irritation.

3.4 Adjusted Strength Preparing System

Guarantee that your solidarity preparing program integrates a fair methodology, focusing on all significant muscle gatherings. This forestalls muscle lopsided characteristics that can prompt wounds.

3.5 Adaptability Preparing

Incorporate ordinary adaptability practices in your daily schedule to work on joint versatility and scope of movement. Yoga and extending schedules can be valuable.

3.6 Rest and Recuperation

Permit adequate time for rest and recuperation between strength instructional meetings. Muscles need time to fix and develop further, decreasing the gamble of abuse wounds.

4. Treatment of Normal Strength Preparing Wounds

4.1 RICE Convention

The RICE convention (Rest, Ice, Pressure, Height) is a typical way to deal with starting treatment for some strength preparing wounds. Rest the impacted region, apply ice to lessen irritation, use pressure to help the harmed region, and hoist it to limit enlarging.

4.2 Torment The board

Over-the-counter pain killers like ibuprofen or acetaminophen might assist with overseeing torment and diminish aggravation. Notwithstanding, talk with a medical services supplier prior to taking any drug.

4.3 Active recuperation

In instances of additional serious wounds, exercise based recuperation might be important. Actual specialists can foster customized practice projects to advance recuperating, reestablish capability, and forestall future wounds.

4.4 R.I.C.E.R.

For specific wounds, particularly injuries and strains, the R.I.C.E.R. convention might be utilized. It incorporates Rest, Ice, Pressure, Rise, and Reference (to a clinical expert) for a more exact finding and treatment plan.

4.5 Rest and Recuperation

Rest is fundamental for recuperating. Give your body satisfactory chance to recuperate prior to continuing strength preparing. Overlooking rest can worsen wounds or lead to constant circumstances.

5. True Applications and Contextual analyses

5.1 Contextual analysis: Forestalling Rotator Sleeve Wounds

A strength preparing devotee saw shoulder inconvenience during above works out. Subsequent to looking for direction from a mentor, they further developed their shoulder portability and procedure, lessening the gamble of rotator sleeve wounds.

5.2 Contextual investigation: Overseeing Low Back Agony

An individual encountering low back torment during squats and deadlifts talked with an actual specialist. They were shown legitimate lifting methods, center reinforcing works out, and got manual treatment to ease torment and further develop structure.

5.3 Contextual investigation: Forestalling Knee Wounds

A sprinter who incorporated strength preparing to further develop execution confronted knee torment during thrusts and squats. They talked with a games physiotherapist, who prescribed designated activities to reinforce the quadriceps and hip muscles, diminishing burden on the knees.

9.2 Injury Prevention Strategies

Wounds can upset day to day existence, prevent actual work, and have long haul outcomes. In any case, numerous wounds are preventable through the execution of successful systems. This exhaustive aide dives into different injury counteraction systems, incorporating individual propensities, wellbeing measures, and proactive measures for various parts of life. By getting it and applying these procedures, people can have more secure and more dynamic existences.

1. **The Significance of Injury Counteraction**

   1.1 Why Injury Counteraction Matters

   Wellbeing and Prosperity: Forestalling wounds guarantees better physical and psychological well-being, empowering people to appreciate life without limit.

   Personal satisfaction: Wounds can restrict portability and support in day to day exercises. Injury counteraction jam personal satisfaction.

   Monetary Effect: Wounds bring about clinical expenses and lost efficiency. Forestalling wounds decreases monetary weights.

Long haul Results: A few wounds make enduring impacts. Injury avoidance can forestall constant agony and handicap.

2. **Injury Anticipation Procedures**

2.1 Individual Wellbeing Propensities

1. **Safe Driving:** Pursuing safe driving routines, complying with transit regulations, and staying away from interruptions can diminish the gamble of engine vehicle mishaps.
2. **Bicycle Security:** Wearing head protectors, utilizing lights, and adhering to traffic guidelines while cycling assist with forestalling bike related wounds.
3. **Walker Security:** Focusing on traffic lights and utilizing crosswalks can limit the gamble of person on foot mishaps.
4. **Liquor and Substance Use:** Keeping away from liquor or medication debilitation while working vehicles or participating in exercises lessens the probability of mishaps.

2.2 Home Wellbeing

1. **Falls Anticipation:** Introducing handrails, utilizing non-slip mats, and keeping walkways clear at home can forestall falls, particularly among the older.
2. **Fire Wellbeing:** Introducing smoke alarms, having fire quenchers, and rehearsing emergency exit plans add to home security.
3. **Childproofing:** Childproofing homes, including getting cupboards, entryways, and plugs, forestalls wounds to small kids.

2.3 Work environment Security

1. **Ergonomics:** Legitimate ergonomics in the work environment, for example, flexible seats and PC screens, can forestall outer muscle wounds.
2. **Individual Defensive Hardware (PPE):** Wearing proper PPE, like head protectors, gloves, or security goggles, in perilous workplaces is fundamental.
3. **Preparing:** Satisfactory preparation in work environment well-being methodology and conventions diminishes the gamble of mishaps and wounds.

2.4 Games and Proactive tasks

1. **Legitimate Gear:** Utilizing great fitted and suitable athletic gear, like protective caps, cushions, and footwear, is significant for injury anticipation.
2. **Warm-Up and Chill Off:** Integrating warm-up and chill off schedules into proactive tasks readies the body and decreases the gamble of wounds.
3. **Method and Structure:** Learning and rehearsing right procedures and structure in sports and proactive tasks can forestall abuse wounds.

2.5 Wellness and Exercise

1. **Continuous Movement:** Advancing step by step in wellness schedules permits the body to adjust securely and lessens the gamble of abuse wounds.
2. **Broadly educating:** Taking part in various activities and exercises forestalls abuse wounds and advances generally speaking wellness.
3. **Rest and Recuperation:** Permitting adequate time for rest and recuperation between exercises is fundamental for forestalling exhaustion related wounds.

III. Kid Injury Counteraction

3.1 Childproofing the Home

Secure Furnishings: Anchor weighty furniture to forestall tip-overs.

Kid Entryways: Introduce doors to confine admittance to steps and other risky regions.

Wellbeing Locks: Use security hooks on cupboards and drawers to keep hazardous things far off.

3.2 Bike Security

Protective cap Use: Guarantee youngsters wear appropriately fitting head protectors while trekking.

Preparing Wheels: Use preparing wheels for youthful cyclists until they foster equilibrium and certainty.

3.3 Jungle gym Security

Surface Material: Pick jungle gyms with shock-retaining surfaces like elastic or wood chips.

Management: Oversee youngsters on jungle gyms to forestall mishaps.

3.4 Vehicle Seat Security

Legitimate Establishment: Guarantee vehicle seats are accurately introduced and proper for the youngster's age and size.

Back Confronting Seats: Keep babies in back confronting vehicle seats until they arrive at the suggested age and weight.

IV. Injury Avoidance for Seniors

4.1 Falls Avoidance

Home Alterations: Make home changes to decrease fall gambles, including introducing get bars and eliminating stumbling dangers.

Strength and Equilibrium Activities: Take part in strength and equilibrium activities to further develop security.

4.2 Drug The board

Drug Audit: Routinely survey prescriptions with medical services suppliers to decrease the gamble of connections or secondary effects.

Drug Capacity: Store prescriptions appropriately to forestall inadvertent harming.

4.3 Normal Tests

Wellbeing Appraisals: Customary exams with medical services suppliers help distinguish and address medical problems early.

Vision and Hearing: Address vision and hearing issues to keep up with situational mindfulness.

V. Sports Injury Counteraction

5.1 Pre-Cooperation Physicals

Clinical Assessment: Pre-cooperation physicals survey a singular's wellness and recognize any basic ailments.

5.2 Legitimate Molding

Strength Preparing: Strength preparing programs custom fitted to explicit games lessen the gamble of wounds.

Adaptability Preparing: Adaptability practices work on joint portability and lessen the gamble of strains and injuries.

5.3 Warm-Up and Chill Off

Dynamic Warm-Up: Integrate dynamic stretches and developments into warm-up schedules.

Cool-Down: Cool down with static stretches to keep up with adaptability and decrease muscle irritation.

VI. Work environment Injury Avoidance

6.1 Ergonomics

Ergonomic Workstations: Plan workstations with customizable seats, consoles, and screen levels to lessen outer muscle strain.

Normal Breaks: Enjoy short reprieves to stand, stretch, and rest the eyes to forestall abuse wounds.

6.2 Preparation and Training

Wellbeing Preparing: Bosses ought to give security preparing and instruction to representatives on work environment dangers and strategies.

Revealing Systems: Lay out clear strategies for detailing security concerns and occurrences.

VII. Sports-Explicit Injury Anticipation

7.1 Soccer

Appropriate Footwear: Guarantee players wear soccer-explicit spikes to forestall slips and falls.

Warm-Up: Incorporate dynamic stretches and ball work in warm-up schedules.

7.2 Ball

Lower leg Backing: Use lower leg supports or tape for added help during focused energy developments.

Bounce Preparing: Consolidate hop preparing to lessen the gamble of knee wounds.

7.3 Running

Legitimate Footwear: Pick running shoes that match your stride and foot type.

Steady Movement: Continuously increment running distance and force to forestall abuse wounds.

9.3 Muscular Strength in Everyday Life

Strong strength is a basic part of actual wellness that assumes a crucial part in regular daily existence. It empowers people to perform different assignments and exercises easily, upgrades by and large prosperity, and adds to a functioning and free way of life. In this exhaustive aide, we will investigate the meaning of solid strength in day to day

existence, its effect on different parts of wellbeing and usefulness, and down to earth applications that feature its significance.

1. **The Meaning of Solid Strength**
   1.1 Meaning of Solid Strength
   Solid strength alludes to the greatest power a muscle or gathering of muscles can apply against obstruction in a solitary exertion. It is normally estimated as far as the most extreme weight an individual can lift for a particular activity or development.
   1.2 The Job of Strong Strength
   Solid strength fills in as the establishment for various day to day exercises and practical developments. It impacts a singular's

capacity to lift, convey, push, pull, and play out many actual undertakings.

2. **Effect of Strong Strength on Day to day existence**

2.1 Useful Autonomy

Keeping up with satisfactory strong strength is fundamental for useful freedom in day to day existence. It empowers people to perform exercises of day to day living (ADLs) like dressing, washing, and getting in and out of seats without help.

2.2 Versatility and Adaptability

Solid strength adds to worked on joint soundness and scope of movement. Solid muscles assist with supporting joints and diminish the gamble of wounds or distress connected with development.

2.3 Injury Anticipation

Having advanced muscles gives added insurance to the body. Solid muscles can assimilate influence powers during falls or mishaps, diminishing the gamble of breaks and wounds.

2.4 Stance and Arrangement

Strong strength in the center, back, and stomach muscles upholds appropriate stance and spinal arrangement. Keeping up with great stance forestalls back torment and related issues.

2.5 Weight The board

Muscle tissue requires more energy (calories) for upkeep than fat tissue. In this way, people with higher bulk will generally have a more effective digestion, making it simpler to oversee body weight and body organization.

3. **Advantages of Solid Strength**

3.1 Better Equilibrium and Security

Solid muscles, especially in the lower body, upgrade equilibrium and soundness. This is particularly significant for exercises like strolling on lopsided territory or exploring steps.

3.2 Improved Bone Wellbeing

Obstruction preparing, which works on strong strength, likewise invigorates bone development and thickness. More grounded bones are less defenseless to breaks and osteoporosis.

3.3 Expanded Metabolic Rate

Muscle tissue has a higher resting metabolic rate than fat tissue. This implies that people with more muscle consume more calories very still, adding to weight the board.

3.4 Improved Cardiovascular Wellbeing

Strength preparing can prompt lower pulse and worked on cardiovascular wellbeing. More grounded muscles additionally lessen the burden on the heart during proactive tasks.

3.5 Mental Prosperity

Normal activity, including strength preparing, has been connected to further developed mind-set, diminished pressure, and improved mental prosperity.

4. **Strong Strength in Regular Exercises**

4.1 Lifting and Conveying

Strong strength is fundamental for lifting and conveying objects, like food, baggage, or furniture. Solid leg and back muscles give the power expected to these errands.

4.2 Climbing Steps

Rising and diving steps require leg strength and equilibrium. Solid strength in the quadriceps, hamstrings, and lower leg muscles assumes a huge part in step climbing.

4.3 Family Tasks

Normal family tasks like vacuuming, wiping, and planting include dreary developments that advantage from solid strength and perseverance.

4.4 Playing with Youngsters

Guardians and parental figures frequently participate in actual play with kids. Solid strength permits grown-ups to partake effectively and securely in exercises like running, playing sports, or lifting youngsters.

4.5 Keeping up with Versatility in Later Years

As people age, keeping up with solid strength turns out to be progressively significant for keeping up with versatility and freedom. Solid muscles lessen the gamble of falls and backing exercises like ascending from a seat or getting in and out of a bath.

5. Reasonable Uses of Strong Strength

5.1 Strength Preparing

Integrating strength preparing practices into a wellness routine is one of the best ways of developing and keep up with solid fortitude. Normal strength preparing practices incorporate squats, deadlifts, seat presses, and columns.

5.2 Bodyweight Activities

Bodyweight practices like push-ups, pull-ups, jumps, and boards are open and require insignificant gear. They can be performed at home or in outside settings.

5.3 Utilitarian Preparation

Utilitarian preparation centers around developments that mirror ordinary exercises. It incorporates practices like squats, jumps, and portable weight swings that further develop strength and portability for day to day errands.

5.4 Obstruction Groups

Obstruction groups are adaptable devices for strength preparing. They give obstruction in different headings, considering designated muscle commitment.

5.5 Adaptability and Versatility Preparing

Integrating adaptability and versatility practices into a wellness routine forestalls muscle uneven characters and upgrades by and large usefulness.

6. Maturing and Solid Strength

6.1 Sarcopenia

Sarcopenia alludes to progress in years related muscle misfortune. It can prompt decreased strength and usefulness. Ordinary strength preparing can help battle sarcopenia and keep up with bulk in more seasoned grown-ups.

6.2 Fall Counteraction

Decreasing the gamble of falls is critical for seniors. Strength preparing programs that target leg and center muscles can upgrade equilibrium and steadiness, diminishing the gamble of falls.

6.3 Freedom

Protecting solid strength in later years improves freedom and personal satisfaction. It permits seniors to keep performing day to day exercises without dependence on guardians.

9.4Muscular Strength and Aging

Maturing is a characteristic piece of life, and it achieves different actual changes in the body. One huge part of maturing is the steady loss of strong strength, a condition known as sarcopenia. Strong strength is a key part of actual wellness that assumes a urgent part in keeping up with generally wellbeing and freedom. In this thorough aide, we will investigate the connection between strong strength and maturing, the effect old enough related muscle misfortune, and procedures for safeguarding and working on solid strength as we become older.

1. **Grasping Strong Strength**

   1.1 Solid Strength Characterized

   Solid strength alludes to the greatest power a muscle or gathering of muscles can apply against obstruction in a solitary exertion. It is commonly estimated as far as the greatest weight an individual can lift for a particular activity or development.

   1.2 The Job of Solid Strength

   Solid strength isn't just about lifting significant burdens; it's fundamental for ordinary exercises and practical freedom. It impacts a singular's capacity to perform undertakings, for example, lifting food, getting up from a seat, and keeping up with equilibrium and security.

2. The Maturing System and Strong Strength

2.1 Sarcopenia: Age-Related Muscle Misfortune

Sarcopenia is a term used to portray the steady loss of bulk and strength that happens with maturing. It normally starts around the age of 30 and advances quickly in later years. Sarcopenia can have huge ramifications for actual capability and generally speaking wellbeing.

2.2 Variables Adding to Sarcopenia

A few variables add to the improvement of sarcopenia:

Hormonal Changes: Age-related hormonal changes, remembering a reduction for testosterone and development chemical levels, can prompt muscle misfortune.

Nourishing Lacks: Deficient protein admission and unfortunate sustenance can debilitate muscle upkeep and fix.

Actual Inertia: A stationary way of life speeds up muscle misfortune and debilitates existing muscles.

Aggravation: Constant irritation can add to muscle squandering.

Neuromuscular Changes: Maturing can influence the nerves that control muscle compressions, prompting diminished muscle capability.

3. Effect of Solid Strength on Maturing

3.1 Practical Autonomy

Keeping up with strong strength is vital for utilitarian freedom as we age. It empowers more seasoned grown-ups to perform exercises of day to day living (ADLs), like dressing, washing, and getting in and out of seats without help.

3.2 Versatility and Equilibrium

Solid strength adds to further developed portability and equilibrium, lessening the gamble of falls and related wounds in more seasoned grown-ups.

3.3 Bone Wellbeing

Strength preparing, which works on strong strength, additionally invigorates bone development and thickness. This is especially significant for lessening the gamble of breaks and osteoporosis in maturing people.

3.4 Metabolic Wellbeing

Muscle tissue has a higher metabolic rate than fat tissue, and that implies that people with more muscle consume more calories very still. Keeping up with or expanding strong strength can assist with overseeing body weight and digestion.

3.5 Cardiovascular Wellbeing

Strength preparing has been connected to bring down pulse and worked on cardiovascular wellbeing. More grounded muscles decrease the burden on the heart during proactive tasks.

4. Procedures for Saving and Working on Solid Strength in Maturing

4.1 Strength Preparing

Integrating strength preparing practices into a standard wellness routine is one of the best ways of developing and keep up with strong fortitude. Opposition practices utilizing free loads, obstruction groups, or weight machines can target explicit muscle gatherings.

4.2 Obstruction Groups

Obstruction groups are flexible instruments for strength preparing. They give obstruction in different bearings, considering designated muscle commitment and giving a protected choice to more seasoned grown-ups.

4.3 Bodyweight Activities

Bodyweight activities, for example, push-ups, squats, rushes, and boards can be performed without the requirement for particular hardware. These activities assist with developing fortitude and further develop muscle perseverance.

4.4 Utilitarian Preparation

Utilitarian preparation centers around developments that emulate regular exercises. Practices like squats, thrusts, and portable weight swings further develop strength and portability for day to day errands.

4.5 Adaptability and Portability

Integrating adaptability and portability practices into a wellness routine forestalls muscle uneven characters and upgrades in general usefulness. Yoga and extending schedules can be valuable for more established grown-ups.

5. **Advantages of Solidarity Preparing in Maturing**

5.1 Protection of Bulk

Customary strength preparing helps protect and possibly increment bulk, countering the impacts of sarcopenia.

5.2 Better Bone Thickness

Obstruction preparing invigorates bone development and keeps up with bone thickness, lessening the gamble of breaks.

5.3 Upgraded Equilibrium and Solidness

Strength preparing practices that focus on the legs and center can altogether further develop equilibrium and steadiness, decreasing the gamble of falls.

5.4 Digestion and Weight The executives

Developing and keeping up with muscle through fortitude preparation adds to a more effective digestion and can assist with overseeing body weight.

5.5 Joint Wellbeing

Strength preparing can assist with supporting joint wellbeing by further developing muscle dependability and decreasing the gamble of wounds connected with outer muscle lopsided characteristics.

6. **Wellbeing Contemplations for More established Grown-ups**

6.1 Counsel with Medical care Suppliers

Prior to starting a strength preparing program, more established grown-ups ought to talk with their medical services suppliers, particularly on the off chance that they have basic ailments.

6.2 Appropriate Structure and Method

Learning and reliably utilizing legitimate structure and method during strength preparing practices is significant to forestall wounds.

6.3 Continuous Movement

Begin with proper opposition levels and steadily increment power to stay away from overexertion and injury.

6.4 Rest and Recuperation

Permit adequate time for rest and recuperation between strength instructional courses to advance muscle fix and lessen the gamble of abuse wounds.

9 788819 666890 7